WEIGHT LOSS
THE VEGAN WAY

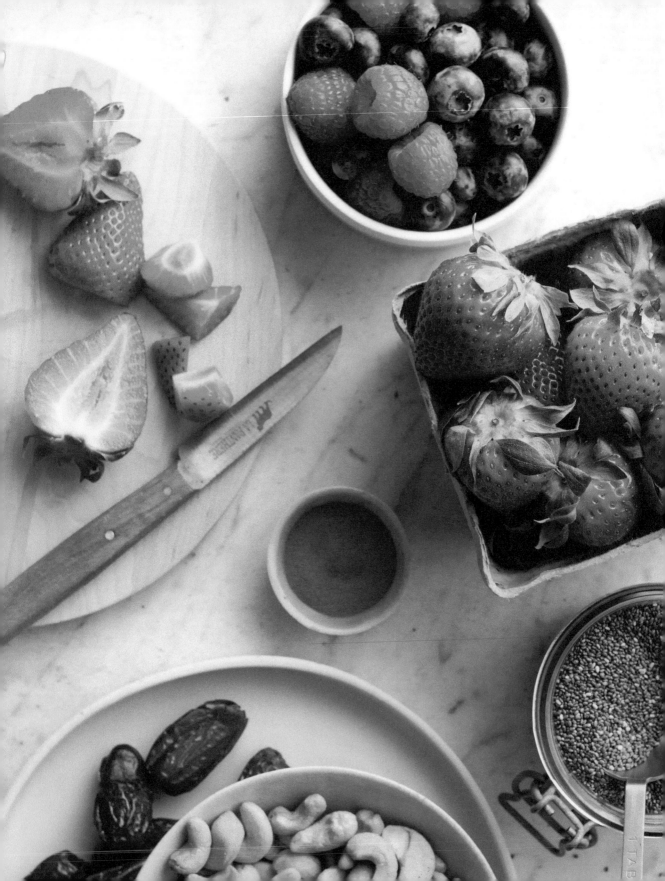

WEIGHT LOSS
THE VEGAN WAY

A 21-Day Meal Plan with Over 75 Easy Recipes

LISA DANIELSON

Photography by Tara Donne

ROCKRIDGE PRESS

For general information on our other products and services or to obtain technical support, please contact our Customer Care Department within the United States at (866) 744-2665, or outside the United States at (510) 253-0500.

Rockridge Press publishes its books in a variety of electronic and print formats. Some content that appears in print may not be available in electronic books, and vice versa.

Interior and Cover Designer: Carlos Esparza
Art Producer: Meg Baggott
Editor: Rachel Feldman
Production Editor: Matthew Burnett

Photography © 2020 Tara Donne. Food styling by Hadas Smirnoff.

Author photograph courtesy of © Maggie Yahvah

Cover: Coconut-Lime Noodle Soup, page 101

ISBN: Print 978-1-64739-344-1 | eBook 978-1-64739-345-8

R0

To all those who believe in being their best selves . . .
little changes add up to big results. Keep at it!

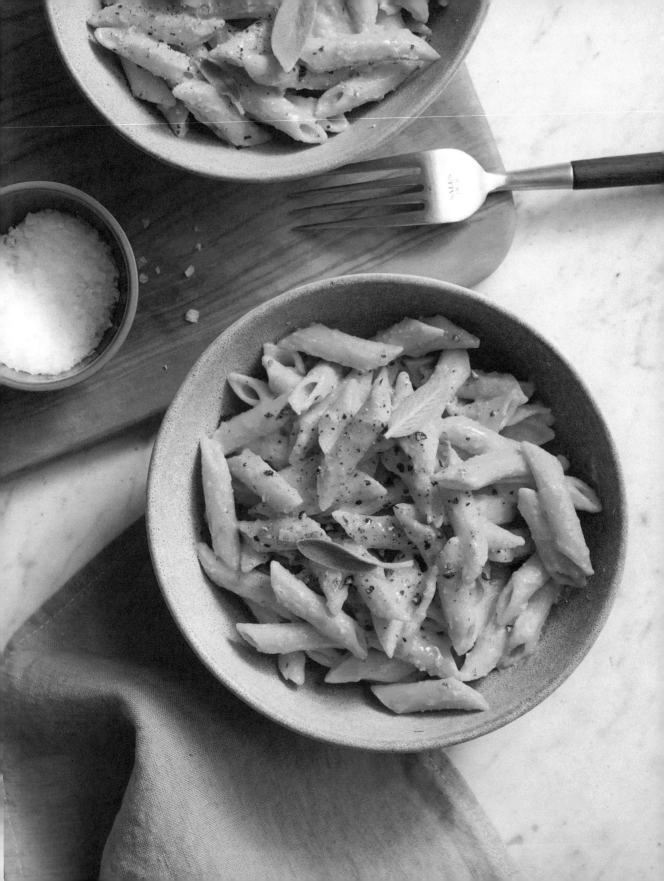

Contents

< Pumpkin-Sage Pasta, page 81

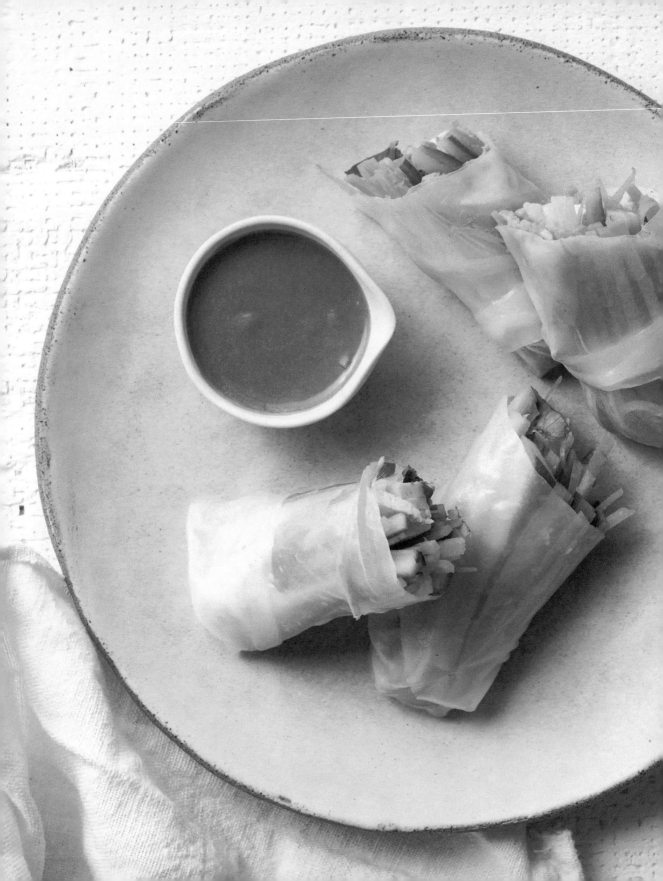

Introduction

My name is Lisa, and I love vegetables. I've been a plant-based eater since I was eight. While I knew early on that meat was not for me, it took me many years to love vegetables.

In my early 20s, I met the man of my dreams and settled into married life. During the course of my first pregnancy, I gained 80 pounds, and even after giving birth to a beautiful baby boy, I had quite a bit of weight to lose. Over the next two years, I lost 60 pounds and finally realized what a balanced diet should look like. Sixteen years (and three more babies) later, I have managed to maintain a healthy, meatless life-style without feeling like I'm sacrificing anything.

The vegan diet has risen in popularity due to groundbreaking documentaries, celebrities, and top athletes all lauding its health results—but it's not just hype. I often hear stories from clients who have tried the vegan diet and have more energy than ever or don't have aches and pains anymore. All of them have lost weight and managed to keep it off. Once you try the vegan way of eating, you'll see food in a new way.

Whether you are a lifelong omnivore or vegan, you will find helpful information and recipes in this book. Weight loss is a difficult journey, but this book will walk you through everything you need to know—and do—to get started.

I hope you're as excited as I am for you to start your journey. This is the beginning of a new, healthier you. Best of luck!

< **Spring Vegetable Rolls with Peanut Sauce, page 76**

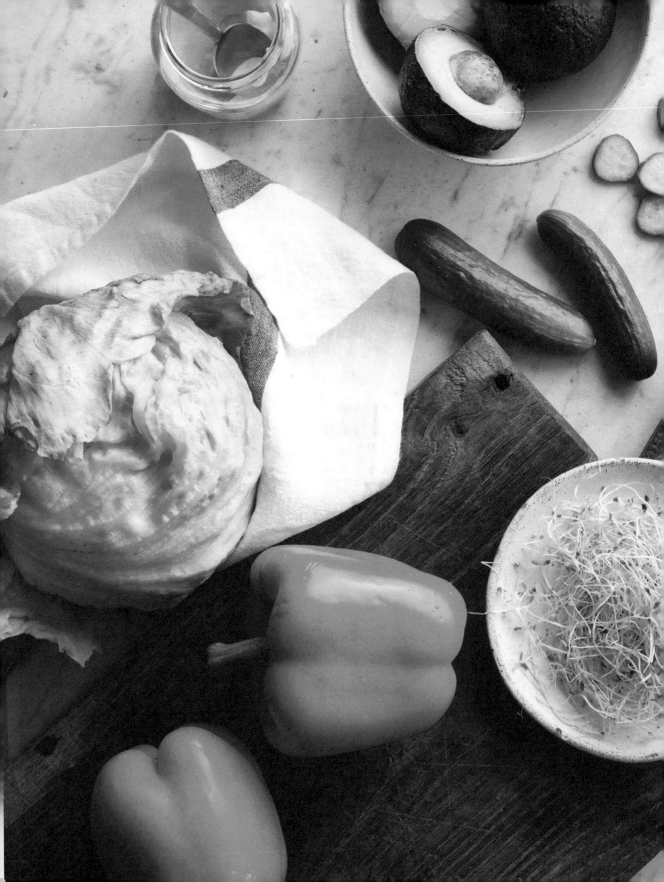

PART ONE

THE VEGAN WAY

First of all, congratulations on taking charge of your health. Whether you've only heard of the vegan diet or you've been eating mostly plant-based foods for a while, you're in the right place; anyone can experience the long list of this diet's health benefits. The best part is that this diet isn't about deprivation—it's about filling your body with a variety of nutrient-dense foods. You'll not only lose weight, you'll also feel reenergized and inspired. My goal is that you will ultimately change your relationship with food for the long term.

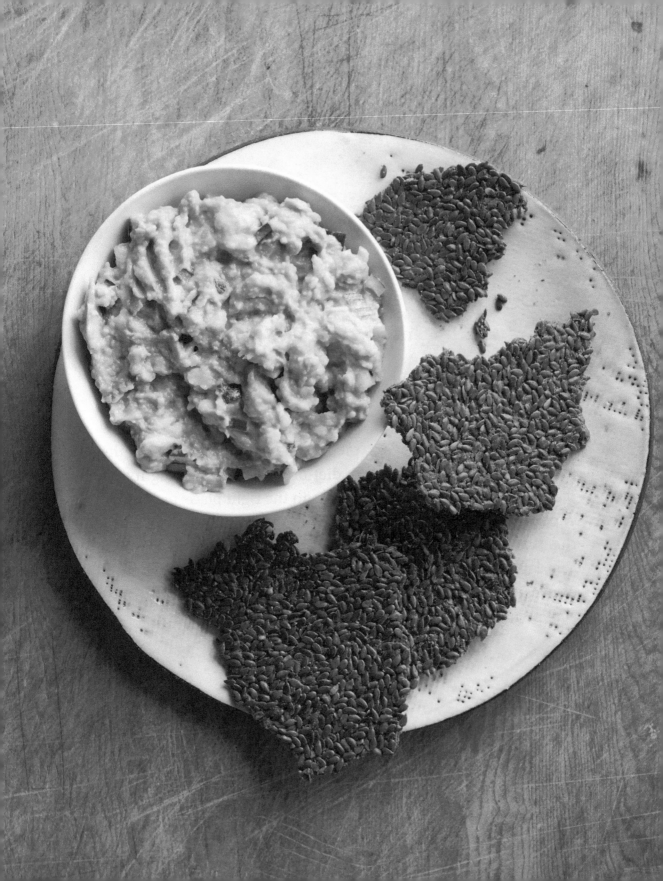

CHAPTER 1

Weight Loss, Powered by Plants

I've been a plant-based eater for more than 32 years, so I know a thing or two about plants! In this chapter, I'll tell you all *you'll* need to know to make informed decisions about your diet. You'll learn why the dieting cycle in America is so flawed, how weight loss really works, and why a vegan diet is the best answer. Learning a bit before jumping in will help give you the confidence needed to succeed.

< Flaxseed Chips and Guacamole, page 108

Your Brain on Dieting

You've probably heard the term "standard American diet" thrown around before; it refers to what the typical American eats daily. But you may not be familiar with the actual makeup of this diet: 63 percent of calories come from refined and processed foods such as soft drinks, potato chips, and packaged foods; 25 percent comes from animal-based products; and 12 percent comes from plant-based sources—half of which are French fries, leaving just a measly 6 percent for real vegetables, nuts, and seeds.

There's a reason the diet is often referred to as "SAD."

There are many factors that contribute to being overweight or obese: genetics, medications, hormones. But the SAD diet is one of the biggest and most preventable reasons. Serious conditions like heart disease and type 2 diabetes have been linked with genetically modified foods, added sugars, and the abundance of refined carbs found in our food. Unfortunately, the things that are the most dangerous for us are also the most accessible—and the most addicting. These foods are so popular *because* of how accessible and addicting they are. They cause your blood sugar to spike—causing a temporary boost in energy and dopamine—and then subsequently crash, leaving you feeling exhausted and in need of another boost. And so, the cycle continues.

Breaking this cycle isn't easy, but it isn't impossible. Educating yourself is the first step.

The Vegan Diet

Plant-based eating, including veganism, is on the rise, and it's no surprise why. Research has shown that a vegan diet can help do the following:

- Promote weight loss
- Reduce the risk of heart disease by lowering cholesterol levels
- Lower the chances of getting certain types of cancer
- Help manage diabetes by lowering A1c levels

Veganism is often considered both a diet and a lifestyle. Many who identify as vegan do not use any animal byproducts for food or other purposes, often due to their personal convictions regarding animal rights or environmental impact. Animal agriculture contributes to 65 percent of global nitrous oxide emissions, 35 to 40 percent of methane emissions, and 9 percent of carbon dioxide emissions, and these are the primary chemicals involved in climate change. Animal agriculture is also known for using a significant amount of water (between 550 and 5,200 gallons of water are used to produce just one pound of beef).

Health is one of the biggest reasons people are turning to the vegan diet today, thanks to all of those aforementioned health benefits. But there is such a thing as an unhealthy vegan diet. You may be avoiding animal products but still consuming mostly packaged, processed foods with added sugars and fats. There are plenty of processed vegan sweets and snacks full of sugar, and vegan meats and cheeses can still be full of salt, soy protein isolates, fat, calories, and various other chemicals.

A healthy vegan diet is rich in vegetables, fruits, legumes, and whole grains. These foods are dense in macronutrients and micronutrients, which help your body function properly. They are high in fiber, antioxidants, B vitamins, and iron. Half of your plate should be vegetables, a quarter should be complex carbs, and a quarter should be a healthy, plant-based protein.

Losing Weight the Vegan Way

So, why do vegans tend to have a lower BMI? A 2013 study comparing the results of non-plant-based and plant-based diets found that vegans lost the most weight over six months—and that's without counting calories. The success was attributed to avoiding saturated fat from meat and cheese and eating plants instead. Here are some more of the specific ways a vegan diet contributes to weight loss.

FILL UP FASTER WITH LESS. According to a 2017 report by the Centers for Disease Control and Prevention (CDC), more than 80 percent of Americans fail to consume the daily recommended amount of fruit or vegetables, missing out on crucial vitamins, minerals, and fiber. Vegetables, which are full of fiber and more nutrient dense than animal-based foods, will help you feel fuller for the cost of far fewer calories. In other words, you can eat more for less calories—more bang for your nutritional buck.

5 STEPS TO WEIGHT LOSS SUCCESS

STEP 1: START SLOW. Just like you wouldn't sign up for a marathon without at least some training, you don't need to jump into the diet or meal plan cold turkey. Maybe spend a week or two making some small, healthy changes first: Remove packaged foods from your diet, drink more water, and opt for vegetarian or vegan proteins if you're currently eating animal products. If you're trying to be more active as well, consider starting by adding a daily 20 minute walk to your routine instead of pushing yourself to spend an hour on the treadmill or in the gym.

STEP 2: DON'T SUFFER. If I could shout one thing from the rooftops, it would be **"DON'T SKIP MEALS OR SNACKS!"** Your body won't function properly or get the nutrients it needs if you decide to skip your meals. Food is fuel, so treat your body right, and you will reap the rewards. And, as we already talked about, not feeding your body enough calories can be just as damaging as eating too much. This step applies to the food you are eating as well; there is nothing worse than hating the food you're eating while on a diet plan. If you find yourself struggling with a dish, here are a few suggestions:

1. If a dish is bland, add some spices or fresh herbs.

2. If you hate mushrooms, don't eat them. Stick with the healthy foods you already know you like. You can add new things from there.

3. At the same time, don't be afraid to try new things. You may find that you really like something new. And who knows—it just may become a staple ingredient in your cooking. What you hated as a child you might like as an adult.

STEP 3: IDENTIFY FOOD BEHAVIOR. Emotional eating is pretty common, but it can range in seriousness. For folks trying to lose weight, it's often a huge obstacle. Emotional eating involves using food to cope with feelings related to anxiety, anger, depression, and even happiness. Try using a food journal to keep track of how you feel when you eat. By recording what you felt and then what/how you ate, some patterns may come to light, and recognizing these patterns may make it easier to practice mindfulness in difficult moments. That way, you can choose to rely on healthier sources of comfort like calling a friend, taking a bath, or going for a walk.

STEP 4: CHANGE YOUR ENVIRONMENT. Creating physical boundaries can be a very strong tool. Is there a place in your house that triggers you to overeat? Particular settings where you find it hard to make healthy food choices? I suggest removing or addressing these barriers as much as possible during the first 21 days. Eat in the main area of your house, specifically around other people. Ask the people you're getting dinner or drinks with to help you make good choices. Make eating nutritious food a positive experience.

STEP 5: CONSISTENCY IS KEY. Studies show that the more consistent someone is with their routine, the more likely they are to make a habit out of it. That's why I created a 21-day meal plan—eating healthy for 21 days will not only help reduce your cravings, it will also empower you to continue making healthy choices.

USE ENERGY FOR OTHER THINGS. A healthy plant-based diet is rich in whole foods and minimizes or avoids processed ingredients like sugar and white flour. The simpler a food is, the easier it is for your body to break it down and digest it. Our bodies were designed to digest plants, allowing for less gas production during digestion, whereas it requires more energy for our bodies to digest animal protein. So, when you eat more plants, your digestive system can take a break, which lets your body direct more energy into being active and repairing muscles.

RECALIBRATE YOUR PALATE. You may know you should be eating more greens and less junk food, but it's hard when you crave foods that are high in sugar and fat. Luckily, you can retrain your palate to enjoy foods that are good for you; it all starts with eliminating the sweet and salty foods you've become accustomed to and trying new, healthy foods. By cutting out the foods we've grown addicted to and eating more vegetables, the palate eventually follows suit. One tip: Try seasoning new foods with familiar flavors you enjoy.

AVOID SATURATED FAT AND CHOLESTEROL. By filling up on fiber, you're also avoiding saturated fat and cholesterol. Consuming less of these icky things contributes to a lower total cholesterol and LDL (bad) cholesterol, lower blood pressure, and lower body mass index (BMI), all of which are associated with longevity and a reduced risk for many chronic diseases.

Weight Loss 101

As a weight loss coach and personal trainer, I help clients navigate the tricky world of losing weight while keeping their sanity intact. I have heard it all when it comes to what people think constitutes healthy weight loss. The truth is that no two people are exactly alike, and thus losing weight can look different for everyone. That said, there are some general guidelines that I'll outline below.

Calorie Intake

Yes, there is a formula to weight loss: expend (burn) more calories each day than you are taking in (eating). The optimal calorie deficit should be large enough to stimulate progressive fat loss, but not so large that you're often hungry. I usually suggest a 250- to 450-calorie deficit from your current daily caloric expenditure; in other words, try eating 250 to 450 fewer calories a day than you usually do.

Counting calories is not a necessary step to losing weight on the vegan diet. But if you are interested in learning more about your body and the process of weight loss, I'd recommend tracking calories for a few weeks until you get a handle on what your portion sizes should be. In order to calculate your daily caloric needs, you'll need to know your **BASAL METABOLIC RATE** (what your body burns at rest).

The easiest way to get this number is by using the Harris-Benedict equation (you can find plenty of websites online that will do the calculating for you after you input your personal numbers):

MEN	BMR = (10 × weight in kg) + (6.25 × height in cm) − (5 × age in years) + 5
WOMEN	BMR = (10 × weight in kg) + (6.25 × height in cm) − (5 × age in years) − 161

Once you find out how many calories you burn at rest, you'll need to multiply that number by your **ACTIVITY FACTOR** (a number based on how active you are). That number should be between 0.2 and 0.5, with 0.2 being a low to moderate level of activity and 0.5 being a high level of activity. Doing that will give you your daily caloric number:

Basal Metabolic Rate × Activity Factor = Daily Caloric Number (maintenance)

Now, this is where I suggest subtracting between 250 and 450 calories from the final number in order to lose weight. Start slow at 250, and if you don't see results after two to three weeks, subtract another 100 calories. The best way to track your calories is by using an app or food journal.

Exercising Regularly

The other way to create a calorie deficit is by burning calories, and increasing your activity helps you do just that. As a certified personal trainer, I help hundreds of people start an exercise program every year. I recommend aiming for at least 150 minutes of moderate exercise per week or 75 minutes of vigorous activity per week, if you're able. Here are some options to consider:

1. **PICK AN EXERCISE THAT YOU ENJOY.** Just like with food, if you hate an exercise, you won't do it. Is it running, walking, aerobic activity, swimming, or biking you like? Pick something that you are excited to do.
2. **JOIN A GYM.** If you don't feel comfortable working out alone, try a group fitness class. It might be a bit intimidating at first, but having a qualified instructor to help guide you along the way will make you feel more confident.
3. **TRY SWIMMING.** If you are unable to start exercising due to an injury or limited mobility, swimming can be a helpful way to get moving. Most local rec centers or YMCAs will have pools and water aerobics classes, as well.
4. **START RESISTANCE TRAINING.** Weight lifting or body weight exercises like push-ups are important because they help build and preserve muscle mass, which burns more calories (so you can eat more!) and helps decrease visceral fat. Visceral fat is the type of fat that surrounds your organs and increases your risk for chronic illness.

Other Lifestyle Changes

While diet and exercise may have the most noticeable impact on weight loss, there are other areas that make a huge difference in overall heath.

MANAGING STRESS

We all have stress in our lives, but chronic and consistent stress can lead to health problems. At the very least, I highly recommend finding healthy outlets for dealing with daily stress. These can range from listening to a podcast, trying a new exercise class, joining a book club, or taking up a relaxing hobby like painting or gardening. There are some great meditation and breathing apps available that may be useful, too.

SLEEPING WELL

Most people need at least seven hours of solid sleep a night, though it varies from person to person. As important as diet and exercise are, sleep is equally as important—and often the most overlooked part of a healthy regimen. Start by trying to get five to six hours of sleep and increase from there. Turn your phone off a few hours before bed to ensure that you can get the deepest sleep possible, especially if you are waking up earlier to work out.

DRINKING WATER

Drinking water is so important to a healthy lifestyle. I suggest drinking at least three-quarters of a gallon (about 96 fluid ounces) of water a day. This will help your body flush out extra carbohydrates that you don't need for fuel. It will also help your digestive system function better and keep you hydrated during your workouts. When you begin to drink more water, you might be running to the bathroom more than usual at first, but soon, your body will regulate itself.

EATING BREAKFAST

Often hailed as the most important meal of the day, breakfast is key to weight loss success. It raises the body's energy level and restores the blood glucose to normal after the overnight fast. Eating breakfast consistently can help your body burn calories more efficiently, leading to faster weight loss.

A Balanced Plate

By now, you know that your meals will mostly consist of vegetables, fruits, and whole grains. A proper balance of all three of these things will be essential to reaching your weight loss goals.

Carbs Are Not the Enemy

Carbs are very important in a healthy diet; they're what our bodies use for energy, fuel, and building and repairing muscle. But not all carbs are created equal.

Refined carbohydrates are the ones found in abundance in processed foods like cakes, crackers, white bread, and breakfast cereals. They may fill you up, but they have little to no nutritional value.

Complex carbohydrates are found in whole grains, beans, sweet potatoes, corn, and beets. These foods help you feel full, staving off the urge to snack. Unrefined, complex carbohydrates include starches and fiber, which have many health benefits.

Plenty of Protein

Not getting enough protein is what scares most people off from trying a vegan diet. Protein is an essential macronutrient, and our bodies need it to function, but it doesn't just come from meat and dairy.

The recommended daily allowance is 0.8 gram of protein per kilogram (2.2 pounds) of body weight for the average adult. So, a person who weighs 150 pounds would need to consume around 61 grams of protein, which is actually pretty easy to do on a vegan diet (note that children, pregnant and nursing mothers, and athletes have different needs, depending on their circumstances). Some examples of plant-based protein include tofu, tempeh, edamame, quinoa, and hemp seeds, though there are plenty more.

Fats in Moderation

Healthy fats provide the body with fatty acids, which it can't generate itself, and they're necessary for absorbing certain vitamins. However, it's important to keep in mind that fats and oils are high in calories and devoid of nutrients themselves, so consuming them in moderation is key. A single serving should usually be about the size of your thumb. Some healthy sources include avocados, tahini, cashews, and chia seeds.

Micronutrients to Consider

Micronutrients are the vitamins and minerals that our bodies require in order to function optimally. A lot of vegetables and a little bit of fruit every day should allow you to garner all the rich vitamins, nutrients, and fiber you need to meet your micronutrient needs. However, vegans can sometimes struggle to get enough of vitamins B_{12} and D, calcium, iron, and iodine.

VITAMIN B_{12} is the only vitamin that plant foods lack, but most plant milks, cereals, and nutritional yeast are fortified with a bioavailable version of B_{12}. If you're not eating these foods daily, a high-quality B_{12} capsule or spray supplement is definitely advisable.

VITAMIN D and calcium are both essential for bone health. Vitamin D isn't found in plant foods or in animals; our bodies make vitamin D by absorbing it from the sun. If you don't live somewhere that is very sunny, take a supplement.

Vitamin D also helps your body absorb **CALCIUM**. Kale and spinach, along with other leafy greens, are fantastic sources of calcium and the most nutrient-dense foods of all.

IRON helps your blood do its job of transporting oxygen throughout the body. Beans and greens are two of the most iron-rich plant foods available; eat them with vitamin C to increase absorption—a little fruit or a bell pepper gives iron an extra boost. Use a cast-iron skillet and cook your greens in a little coconut or olive oil to increase iron absorption.

IODINE is important for thyroid function and makes hormones that keep your metabolism revved up. The easiest way to get iodine is through iodized salt, but you can also find it in kelp, sea vegetables, cranberries, and potatoes.

─────────────────── **KEEPING TRACK** ───────────────────

LOG YOUR FOOD. This doesn't have to be forever, but even if you track your calories for about two to three weeks, you will get a better idea of how much you're consuming. Consider it a mini education. MyFitnessPal is an app that allows you to track your calories by entering your food from a master database.

LOG YOUR STEPS. Shoot for 10,000 steps a day. You can go as simple as a normal pedometer, which is just a few dollars at the store, or you can splurge on a Fitbit or Apple Watch. Make 10,000 steps a day the minimum amount to aim for. If you find yourself consistently under 10,000, it's time to get more active.

LOG YOUR WEIGHT. I suggest you weigh yourself just once a week and enter your weight into an app such as Lose It! or Weight Tracker. This will give you a graph of where you are in relation to your goals. Weighing yourself more frequently can create an unhealthy focus on your weight fluctuations. By tracking your weight only once a week, you can gauge progress without creating an unhealthy balance.

Your Vegan Kitchen

Studies have shown that people who focus on changing their surroundings are more successful at sticking to their diet and losing weight. Overhauling the kitchen is the first step!

MVP Tools and Equipment

HIGH-POWERED BLENDER. A good blender is worth its weight in gold. You can use it to make anything from smoothies and soups to sauces and dips.

FOOD PROCESSOR. Many recipes in this book use a food processor for prep work. This versatile tool will help you puree, chop, and blend.

SALAD SPINNER. Greens are much more affordable when purchased as full heads versus prewashed and bagged lettuces. Salad spinners are useful because after you chop the lettuce, you can wash it, bag it, and store it in your refrigerator.

SHARP KNIVES. One of the many upsides to going vegan is your knife skills will improve. You will be chopping something at just about every meal you make. Having knives of all sizes will help when you are chopping different fruits and vegetables.

SPIRALIZER. You will want to be able to make veggie noodles. Not only are they low-carb, but you can also spiralize anything from zucchini and carrots to sweet potato and yellow squash.

VEGETABLE PEELER. You will use this pretty much every day.

New Ingredients to Try

ARROWROOT. This all-natural powder made from various tuber plants helps thicken soups and sauces.

CHIA SEEDS. These tiny whole grain seeds are high in omega-3s and pack a big nutritional punch. They can be used as a topping or even made into pudding.

CHICKPEA FLOUR. Also referred to as bean flour, chickpea flour is simply ground up dried chickpeas (garbanzo beans). It is high in protein as well as gluten-free.

COCONUT AMINOS. Often used as a substitute for soy sauce, coconut aminos are a salty and buttery condiment derived from coconut sap and sea salt.

EDAMAME. This young, immature soybean contains a high amount of protein. They are mostly served steamed and salted in the pod, though you can buy them fresh or frozen out of the pod, as well.

LAVASH. This unleavened bread, found mostly in Eastern Europe, is popular to serve with Indian food and is an excellent choice for making wraps and pizzas.

LEMONGRASS PASTE. Adding a tablespoon or two of this paste made from ground up lemongrass gives soups, stews, and curries a light lemony flavor. Lemongrass and lemongrass paste are used extensively in Asian cuisine.

NUTRITIONAL YEAST. This is a deactivated yeast that has a cheesy and nutty taste. It's high in protein and B vitamins. It's great for adding to soups and salads and for making vegan cheese.

PEANUT BUTTER POWDER. Dry roasted peanuts are crushed to a powder and the oils are pressed out. Peanut butter powder can be used in recipes on its own or mixed with water to make a sauce.

SHIRATAKI NOODLES. These Japanese noodles are made with Asian yams. They're a great low-calorie, carb-free swap for regular noodles.

STEVIA. This all-natural sweetener comes from a plant called *Stevia rebaudiana*, which has been used in South America for centuries. It is now a mainstream calorie-free sweetener in the United States.

VEGAN PROTEIN POWDER. Made from plant sources such as brown rice, coconut, or hemp, vegan protein powder is usually naturally sweetened and tends to bake better than whey powders.

Preparing for Success

One of the best ways to make healthy eating easier is to be prepared. Beyond following the meal plan in chapter 2, here are some ways you can help yourself stick to a healthy routine.

Meal Plan

You can plan out most of your meals for the week. Start by inspecting your pantry and refrigerator. What ingredients do you already have on hand? After taking inventory, pick out a couple of recipes that excite you and that reuse ingredients to minimize leftovers.

Meal Prep

You don't have to get crazy by prepping all of your meals for the week, but prepping a couple of meals ahead of time will definitely help you stay on track. Prepare overnight oats for breakfast, mason jar salads for lunch, and make two recipes that can be stored in containers ready to reheat for a fast dinner.

Batch Cook

If you're not a huge fan of planning or prepping a lot of meals ahead of time, start with batch cooking. Cook up some beans and grains, prep and roast some vegetables, make a couple sauces—and voila, you'll have food and flavor at your fingertips all week. In part 2, you'll find recipes for batch cook basics and homemade staples. Use these recipes to make other dishes in the book or to throw together your own dishes, like the following examples:

- Perfect Quinoa (page 122) + leafy salad greens + Sweet Potato Steaks (page 126) + Green Goddess Dressing (page 142)

- Easy Lentils (page 121) + Quick and Easy Pickled Cabbage (page 129) + Lemon Tahini Dressing (page 141) + ½ avocado

- Refried Beans (page 120) + Coconut Cilantro Rice (page 127) + chopped romaine lettuce + Not-So-Spicy Jalapeño Hummus (page 144) + sliced red peppers + corn

Ready for Change

Change is hard, but it doesn't have to be as hard as you think. The most important thing is that you're ready to make a change, and the fact that you've picked up this book is a great start. Maybe you're not ready to dive right into the plan. It's okay to start slow; maybe cut out sugary drinks and start incorporating some of the recipes in part 2 into your diet, and then go for the plan. Or maybe you're ready to jump right in. Either way, go at your own pace, and remember that any change at all is a step in the right direction.

Whenever you're ready to make a big change, the 21-day meal plan in chapter 2 will take all of the guesswork out of it. Your meals will be planned for 21 days, and you'll get weekly shopping lists and prep instructions. The meals themselves are great for vegan newbies—easy and tasty.

And beyond the meal plan, whether or not you keep eating vegan, I highly encourage you to keep using the recipes in part 2 to fuel your new, healthier life.

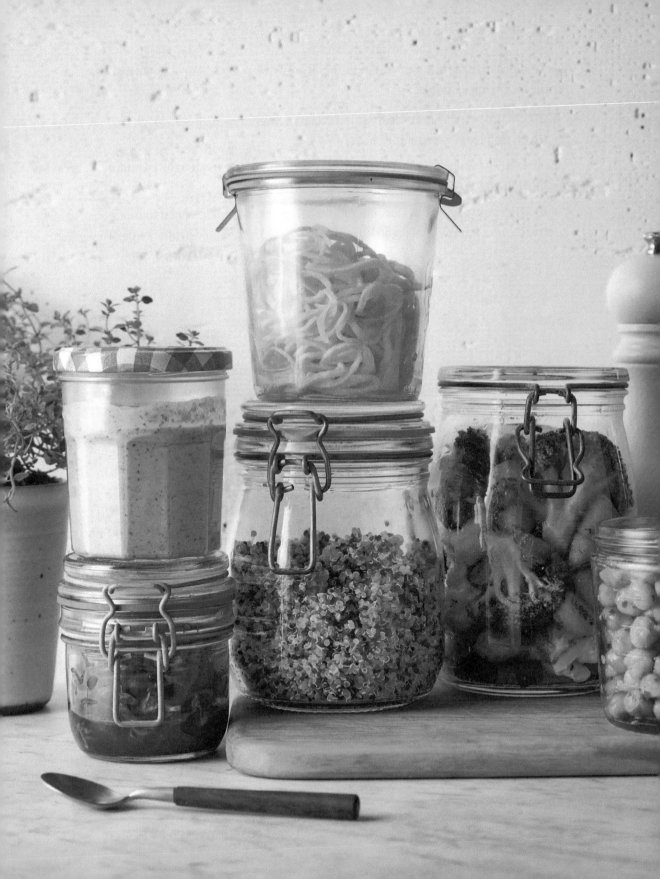

Your 21-Day Meal Plan

This chapter contains your road map to reaching the goals you established in chapter 1. Here, you'll find a 21-day meal plan with shopping lists and prep instructions. Part 2 contains all of the recipes for your 21-day meal plan, plus additional recipes to help you keep eating healthy long after the 21 days.

Managing Expectations

Everyone's weight loss journey looks different. We all have different genetics and predispositions and, therefore, different needs and results. Often in the first week or two of a diet, people will drop a dramatic amount of water weight, but after things start to level out a bit, half a pound a week is a healthy and realistic weight loss goal to set. Slow and steady will always win the race in the weight loss world.

If you're not noticing results, consider whether you're eating too few or too many calories. Eating too few can push your body into starvation mode, where it hangs on to every single ounce. If you're not keeping track of what you're eating, you may be consuming more calories than you even realize. Finding the right calorie intake may require some trial and error.

As always, consult your doctor before starting a new diet and make sure they're on the same page with you about what—and how much—you're consuming.

Notes on the Plan

This meal plan is 21 days long, designed for one person, and created with the goal of weight loss and overall health in mind. The meals for each day come out to about 1,200–1,400 calories. You may need more calories if you're exercising or have landed at a higher calorie intake using the formula on page 9. If that's the case, be sure to add an extra protein-packed snack or smoothie each day. As I've been saying all along, be sure to consult your doctor and take your own special needs into consideration before starting the plan. It is also designed to make things as easy as possible without making the meals feel overly boring or painful. You'll be doing some prep work and maximizing leftovers to make this possible.

Timing

These plans were created with a typical nine-to-five schedule in mind, which is why the majority of prep occurs on Sunday. Note that you'll find the ingredients to make Sunday dinner for Weeks 1 and 2 in the subsequent week (in other words, the ingredients for Sunday's dinner in Week 1 will be in the shopping list for Week 2), since this plan assumes you'll be doing your shopping on the weekends. However, this plan is easy enough that it can work with any schedule. Just take a look at the week and shift the meals and prep work as needed.

Food Storage

- Store prepped and chopped vegetables in sealed containers in the refrigerator.
- Store herbs based on their type:
  - Tender herbs such as parsley, cilantro, dill, and mint should be stored in a glass jar filled with one inch of water in the refrigerator. Cover the top of the herbs with a plastic bag secured with a rubber band.
  - Sturdy herbs such as thyme, rosemary, chives, and sage should be rolled up in damp paper towels, placed in a large zip-top bag, and stored in the refrigerator.
  - Basil should be stored at room temperature.

Cravings

If you have a craving, it is probably your brain signaling that it needs energy or that you are dehydrated. First, drink 12 ounces of water, wait 10 minutes, and see if you are still hungry. If you are still hungry, opt for one of the following fat-fueled snacks:

- Celery with Not-So-Spicy Jalapeño Hummus (page 144)
- ¼ cup of unsalted nuts
- Granola Pumpkin Seed Bars (page 113)
- Half an avocado with Everything Bagel Seasoning (page 140)
- Apples with almond butter

Stocking Your Pantry

The shopping lists for each week include only fresh ingredients, not general pantry staples. To see what pantry staples you'll need to have on hand for each week, consult the "Stocking the Pantry" table on the next page.

Stocking the Pantry

	WEEK 1	WEEK 2	WEEK 3
FATS, OILS, AND VINEGARS			
AVOCADO OIL		X	
COCONUT OIL	X	X	X
NONSTICK COOKING SPRAY			X
OLIVE OIL	X	X	X
SESAME OIL		X	
VINEGAR, RICE WINE		X	
VINEGAR, WHITE	X		
GRAINS AND LEGUMES			
BLACK BEANS, CANNED	X		X
CHICKPEAS, CANNED	X	X	X
LENTILS		X	
OATS, OLD FASHIONED		X	X
OATS, QUICK			X

	WEEK 1	WEEK 2	WEEK 3
QUINOA, MULTICOLORED		X	X
BROTHS, CONDIMENTS, ETC.			
ALMOND MILK, UNSWEETENED	X	X	X
COCONUT MILK, LIGHT	X		X
MUSTARD, DIJON	X		
NUTRITIONAL YEAST		X	X
SOY SAUCE, LOW-SODIUM		X	X
TAHINI	X	X	X
VEGETABLE BROTH, LOW-SODIUM	X		X
NUTS AND SEEDS			
ALMOND BUTTER			X
ALMONDS, RAW	X	X	
CASHEWS, RAW	X	X	
CHIA SEEDS	X	X	X

Continued>

Stocking the Pantry (continued)

	WEEK 1	WEEK 2	WEEK 3
PEANUT BUTTER			X
POPCORN KERNELS	X		
SESAME SEEDS		X	X
DRIED SPICES			
BASIL		X	
CAYENNE PEPPER, GROUND			X
CHILI POWDER	X		
CINNAMON, GROUND	X	X	X
CUMIN, GROUND	X		
CURRY POWDER	X		
GARAM MASALA	X		
GARLIC POWDER	X	X	X
GARLIC SALT		X	
ONION POWDER	X		X

	WEEK 1	WEEK 2	WEEK 3
OREGANO	X	X	
PAPRIKA	X		
PEPPER, BLACK	X	X	X
RED PEPPER FLAKES		X	X
SALT	X	X	X
SEA SALT		X	
TURMERIC, GROUND	X		
POWDERS AND FLOURS			
BAKING POWDER		X	
CHICKPEA FLOUR		X	
PROTEIN POWDER, VANILLA, VEGAN	X		X
SWEETENERS			
COCONUT SUGAR	X		X
STEVIA, LIQUID		X	X

Week 1

Welcome to the first week of the rest of your life! You might feel your energy ebb and flow the first week or two, but know that this is normal and the best thing you can do is stick with the plan and stay consistent. You got this.

A few general rules I like to give my clients:

1. Don't expect perfection right off the bat.
2. Make sure you are getting plenty of sleep, drinking enough water, and staying active through this process.
3. Prep your meals ahead of time—it's crucial to your success.

As I mentioned in the meal plan notes, the shopping ingredients for the Green Goddess Buddha Bowl you'll be eating for dinner on Sunday night are on the shopping list for Week 2. You may have some curry and popcorn leftover, but they'll last in the freezer/pantry for a while. Leftovers are shown in the menu as (LO).

	BREAKFAST	LUNCH	DINNER	SNACK
MONDAY	Blueberry-Lemon Smoothie (page 43)	Chickpea Salad Pinwheels (page 75)	Slow Cooker Sweet Potato Curry (page 96)	1 cup red grapes and ¼ cup almonds
TUESDAY	Blueberry-Lemon Smoothie	Chickpea Salad Pinwheels (LO)	Slow Cooker Sweet Potato Curry (LO)	1 cup red grapes and ¼ cup almonds
WEDNESDAY	Blueberry-Lemon Smoothie	Chickpea Salad Pinwheels (LO)	Slow Cooker Sweet Potato Curry (LO)	1 cup red grapes and ¼ cup almonds
THURSDAY	Southwest Scrambled "Eggs" (page 54)	Chickpea Salad Pinwheels (LO)	Cauliflower Tacos (page 94)	2 cups Churro Popcorn (page 114)
FRIDAY	Southwest Scrambled "Eggs" (LO)	Slow Cooker Sweet Potato Curry (LO)	Cauliflower Tacos (LO)	2 cups Churro Popcorn
SATURDAY	Southwest Scrambled "Eggs" (LO)	Slow Cooker Sweet Potato Curry (LO)	Cauliflower Tacos (LO)	2 cups Churro Popcorn
SUNDAY	Southwest Scrambled "Eggs" (LO)	Cauliflower Tacos (LO)	Green Goddess Buddha Bowl (page 90)	1 cup Churro Popcorn

Buy This

FRUITS AND VEGETABLES

- Avocado (1)
- Bananas (2)
- Bell peppers, red (2)
- Blueberries, fresh or frozen (18 ounces)
- Carrots (3 large)
- Cauliflower (1 head)
- Celery (1 stalk)
- Coleslaw, raw (14 ounces)
- Grapes, red (for snacking, about 1 pound)
- Lemons (3)
- Lime (1)
- Onion, white (1)
- Onion, yellow (1)
- Radishes (3)
- Spinach (10 ounces)
- Sweet potatoes (4 medium)

FRESH SPICES AND HERBS

- Garlic (1 head)

PROTEIN

- Tofu, extra-firm lite (28 ounces)

WEEKLY CANNED, DRIED, AND PACKAGED GOODS

- Pumpkin puree, 1 (29-ounce) can
- Tortillas, whole grain, 8-inch (4)
- Tortillas, corn, 6-inch (8)

Prep This

1. Prep the Blueberry-Lemon Smoothie by filling sandwich-size zip-top bags with all of the ingredients except the protein powder and almond milk. Place the bags in the freezer. When you're ready to make the smoothie, remove a smoothie bag from the freezer and let it thaw on the counter for about 5 minutes before adding the rest of the ingredients.
2. Make the Chickpea Salad Pinwheels and store them in the refrigerator.
3. Prep all of the vegetables for the Slow Cooker Sweet Potato Curry. On Monday morning, add all of the ingredients to the slow cooker before you leave for work or errands. Otherwise, cook it in a regular pot on Monday evening. Portion out 5 servings for the week and freeze the rest of the curry. I like to store curries, soups, and stews in gallon-size zip-top bags, which I lay flat in the freezer for easy stacking. If you prefer, serve the curry with riced cauliflower or zoodles.

ON WEDNESDAY

1. If you have a bit more time in the mornings, you can opt to make the Southwest Scrambled "Eggs" right before eating. For those shorter on time, make the "eggs" tonight and store them in the refrigerator.
2. Make half a batch of the Churro Popcorn.

Week 2

Great job making it through Week 1! The first week can often be the most challenging part of trying something new. But the good news is you probably learned a few things about yourself and hopefully are starting to feel a bit better. Week 2 is where you will mostly see the benefits of eating a plant-based diet really pay off. Expect to have more energy and feel less sluggish. The meal plan for this week is simple, yet the dishes are super flavorful. Enjoy!

	BREAKFAST	LUNCH	DINNER	SNACK
MONDAY	Power Muesli (page 45)	Edamame and Snow Pea Power Salad (page 61)	Green Goddess Buddha Bowl (LO)	⅓ cup Roasted Chickpeas, Four Ways (page 106)
TUESDAY	Power Muesli	Edamame and Snow Pea Power Salad (LO)	Green Goddess Buddha Bowl (LO)	⅓ cup Roasted Chickpeas, Four Ways
WEDNESDAY	Power Muesli	Edamame and Snow Pea Power Salad (LO)	Green Goddess Buddha Bowl (LO)	⅓ cup Roasted Chickpeas, Four Ways
THURSDAY	Power Muesli	Edamame and Snow Pea Power Salad (LO)	Easy Marinara Lentils (page 86)	1 rice cake with ¼ avocado
FRIDAY	Spring Vegetable Muffins (page 55)	Easy Marinara Lentils (LO)	Superfood Pesto Zoodles (page 80)	1 rice cake with ¼ avocado
SATURDAY	Spring Vegetable Muffins	Superfood Pesto Zoodles (LO)	Easy Marinara Lentils (LO)	1 rice cake with ¼ avocado
SUNDAY	Spring Vegetable Muffins	Easy Marinara Lentils (LO)	Thai-Inspired Coconut Curry (page 98)	1 rice cake with ¼ avocado

Buy This

FRUITS AND VEGETABLES

- Asparagus (1 bunch or 9 ounces)
- Avocado (1)
- Bell pepper, red (1)
- Blackberries (6 ounces)
- Broccoli (2 pounds)
- Cabbage, purple, raw (1 head), or pickled, 1 (24-ounce) jar
- Dates, Medjool, pitted (4)
- Edamame, shelled, frozen (1½ pounds)
- Greens for salad (4 cups)
- Lemon (1)
- Onion, green (1)
- Onion, red (1)
- Radishes (6)
- Snow peas (1 pound)
- Spinach (5 ounces)
- Sweet potato (2)
- Tomatoes, cherry (1 pint)
- Vegetables for roasting: broccoli, cauliflower, rainbow carrots, asparagus, or Brussels sprouts (choose 4, 1 bunch each)
- Zucchini (2), or 10 ounces pre-spiralized zucchini noodles

FRESH SPICES AND HERBS

- Basil (2 bunches)
- Garlic (1 head)
- Parsley (1 bunch)

WEEKLY CANNED, DRIED, AND PACKAGED GOODS

- Canned tomatoes, San Marzano, 2 (28-ounce) cans
- Rice cakes, 1 (4.47-ounce) bag

Prep This

1. Prep 4 servings of the Power Muesli. Store them in the refrigerator.
2. Cook a batch of Perfect Quinoa (page 122) for the Edamame and Snow Pea Power Salad and the Green Goddess Buddha Bowl. Finish making the salad and store 4 individual portions in separate containers in the refrigerator.
3. Make the Roasted Chickpeas, Four Ways (any savory variation).
4. Make the remaining components for the Green Goddess Buddha Bowl, doubling the batch. Note that one batch of the Green Goddess Dressing will suffice for four servings of the salad. Assemble a bowl for dinner tonight, then store the rest of the components separately in the refrigerator.

ON THURSDAY

1. Make the Spring Vegetable Muffins. Once they are cooled, store them in a sealed gallon-size zip-top bag in the refrigerator. These can be reheated in the microwave at 50 percent power for 1 minute.
2. Make a double batch of Easy Marinara Lentils for dinner. Store the leftovers for the rest of the week in the refrigerator. Triple the batch of Vegan Parmesan so that one batch can be used in the Superfood Pesto Zoodles on Friday night.

Week 3

Two weeks down—nicely done! You probably feel like you're getting into a rhythm. You have all the tools you need and the recipes in part 2 to keep you going, so I encourage you to keep up the momentum and continue on to a fourth week. This week includes some great staple recipes that you will want to make over and over. Again, don't forget the importance of prepping your meals ahead of time. I know it can take some organization to plan and prep the food, but it will save your sanity in the end. Good luck!

	BREAKFAST	LUNCH	DINNER	SNACK
MONDAY	Spring Green Detox Smoothie (page 42)	Kale Caesar Salad (page 62)	Thai-Inspired Coconut Curry (LO)	2 Lemon-Chia Powerbites (page 116)
TUESDAY	Spring Green Detox Smoothie	Kale Caesar Salad (LO)	Thai-Inspired Coconut Curry (LO)	2 Lemon-Chia Powerbites
WEDNESDAY	Spring Green Detox Smoothie	Kale Caesar Salad (LO)	Tex-Mex Enchilada Bake (page 92)	2 Lemon-Chia Powerbites
THURSDAY	Spring Green Detox Smoothie	Kale Caesar Salad (LO)	Pad Thai (page 83)	1 cup Kale Chips (page 104)
FRIDAY	Quick Apple-Cinnamon Oatmeal (page 48)	Tex-Mex Enchilada Bake (LO)	Pad Thai (LO)	1 cup Kale Chips
SATURDAY	Quick Apple-Cinnamon Oatmeal (LO)	Tex-Mex Enchilada Bake (LO)	Pad Thai (LO)	1 cup Kale Chips
SUNDAY	Quick Apple-Cinnamon Oatmeal (LO)	Pad Thai (LO)	Tex-Mex Enchilada Bake (LO)	1 cup Kale Chips

Buy This

FRUITS AND VEGETABLES

- Apple, red (1)
- Bell pepper, red (3)
- Broccoli (1 head)
- Carrots (9)
- Cauliflower, riced (3 cups)
- Kale, curly (3 bunches)
- Lemons (4)
- Limes (2)
- Onion, white (2)
- Oranges (2)
- Potatoes, Yukon Gold (8)
- Scallions (4)
- Snap peas (3 cups)
- Spinach (15 ounces)

FRESH HERBS AND SPICES

- Cilantro (2 bunches)
- Garlic (1 head)
- Ginger (1-inch piece)

WEEKLY CANNED, DRIED, AND PACKAGED GOODS

- Brown rice noodles, 1 (8-ounce) package
- Coconut flakes, unsweetened, 1 (7-ounce) bag
- Corn, 1 (15.25-ounce) can
- Enchilada sauce, low-sodium, 1 (15-ounce) can
- Red curry paste, 1 (4-ounce) jar
- Tomatoes, fire-roasted, 1 (14-ounce) can

Prep This

1. Prep the Spring Green Detox Smoothie by filling sandwich-size zip-top bags with all of the ingredients except the protein powder and almond milk. Place the bags in the freezer. When you're ready to make the smoothie, remove a smoothie bag from the freezer and let it thaw on the counter for about 5 minutes before adding the rest of the ingredients.
2. Prep a batch of Roasted Chickpeas (any savory variation) and a batch of Lemon Tahini Dressing for the Kale Caesar Salad. Combine the kale and the dressing in 4 separate containers for the week. Pack the chickpeas separately.
3. Make the Thai-Inspired Coconut Curry. Eat 1 serving for dinner and store the rest in the refrigerator for the week.
4. Make the Lemon-Chia Powerbites.

ON WEDNESDAY

1. Make the Tex-Mex Enchilada Bake. Eat 1 serving and store the rest in the refrigerator for the week.
2. Make a batch of Kale Chips to snack on the rest of the week.

ON THURSDAY

1. If you don't have time to cook in the morning, prepare the Quick Apple-Cinnamon Oatmeal tonight.

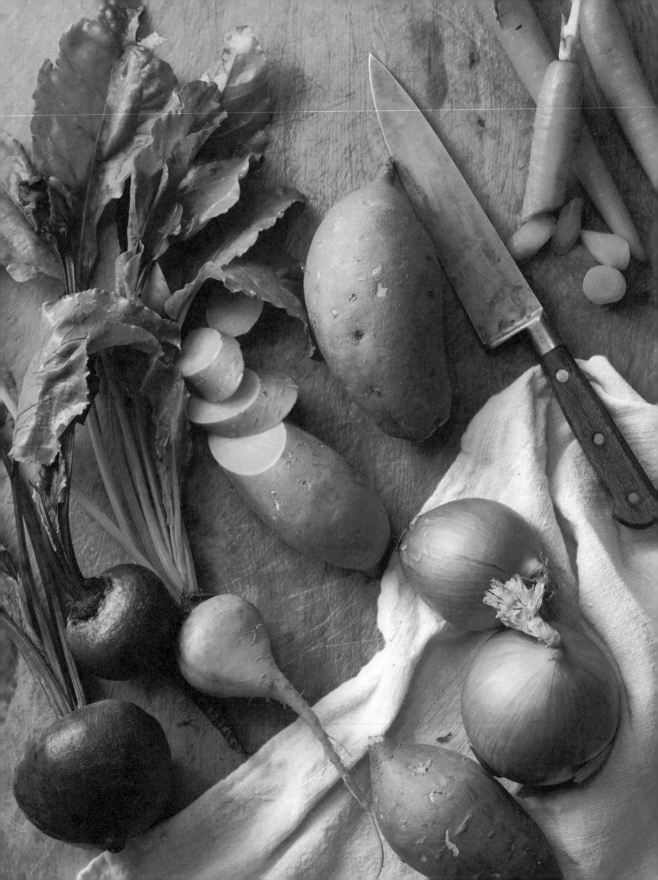

PART TWO

HEALTHY VEGAN RECIPES

The recipes in this book are optimized for health and weight loss, but that doesn't mean they sacrifice ease or flavor. My goal was to show-case the diversity and deliciousness of the vegan diet as well as to prove that anyone can cook vegan! You'll see specific labels that highlight attributes of the recipe:

5-Ingredient (recipe uses 5 ingredients total [aside from pantry staples, such as oils])

Gluten-Free (doesn't use gluten-containing ingredients)

No Cook (recipe doesn't require cooking)

Nut-Free (doesn't use nuts or nut byproducts)

One Pot (recipe only takes one main piece of equipment to make, such as one pot, one skillet, one pan, or one baking dish)

Quick (dishes that can be made in fewer than 30 minutes)

Soy-Free (doesn't use any ingredients that contain soy)

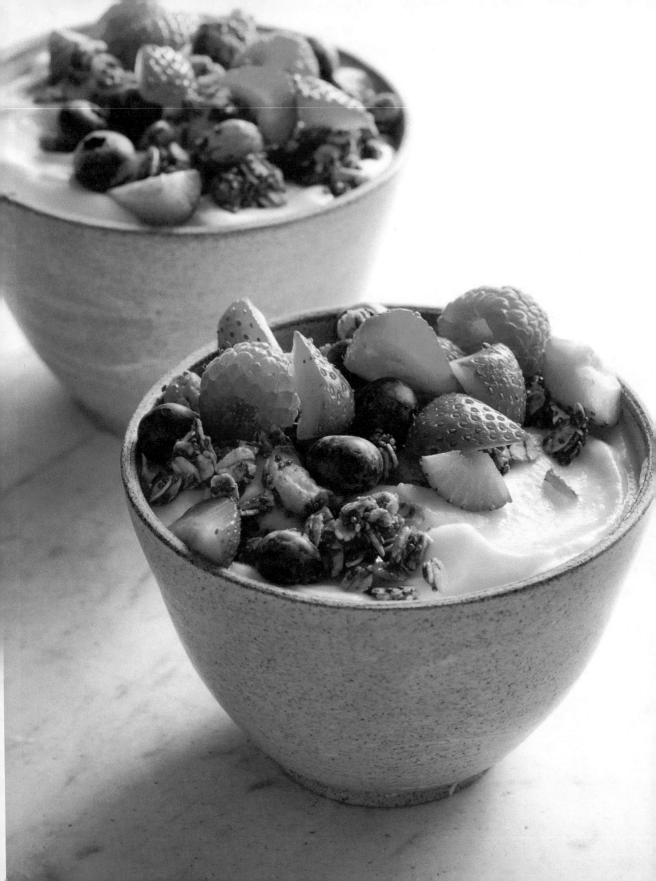

CHAPTER 3

Breakfasts and Beverages

< **Triple Berry Coconut Parfait, page 51**

Spring Green Detox Smoothie

Prep time: 5 minutes / Serves 1

QUICK

NO COOK

GLUTEN-FREE

½ cup unsweetened
   almond milk

2½ tablespoons (1 scoop)
   vegan protein powder

1½ cups chopped spinach

½ medium
   orange, peeled

¼ lemon, peel on

2 tablespoons chia seeds

5 ice cubes

In a high-powered blender, add the almond milk, protein powder, spinach, orange, lemon, chia seeds, and ice cubes and blend on high speed for 1 minute.

Ingredient tip: Leaving the peel on the lemon might seem a bit funny, but the peel adds flavor and essential vitamins for a nutritional boost. The peel has the highest concentration of antioxidants, which helps the liver detoxify the body.

Make ahead: To prep your smoothies ahead of time, fill sandwich-size zip-top bags with all the ingredients except the protein powder and almond milk. Store them in the freezer for up to four weeks. To use, place one bag of ingredients in a blender, add the protein powder and almond milk, and blend on high until smooth.

Smart shopping: I recommend IdealRaw Vanilla Protein Powder, which is vegan and doesn't contain any artificial sweeteners.

Per serving: Calories: 303; Fat: 14g; Protein: 22g; Carbohydrates: 25g; Fiber: 14g; Sugar: 9g

Blueberry-Lemon Smoothie

Prep time: 5 minutes / Serves 1

1 cup unsweetened
  almond milk

2½ tablespoons (1 scoop)
  vegan protein powder

1 cup frozen blueberries

¼ lemon, peel on

1 teaspoon chia seeds

½ banana, frozen

5 ice cubes

In a high-powered blender, add the almond milk, protein powder, blueberries, lemon, chia seeds, banana, and ice cubes and blend on high speed for 1 minute.

QUICK

NO COOK

GLUTEN-FREE

Ingredient tip: Leaving the peel on the lemon might seem a bit funny, but the peel adds flavor and essential vitamins for a nutritional boost. The peel has the highest concentration of antioxidants, which helps the liver detoxify the body.

Make ahead: To prep your smoothies ahead of time, fill sandwich-size zip-top bags with all the ingredients except the protein powder and almond milk. Store them in the freezer for up to four weeks.

Smart shopping: I recommend IdealRaw Vanilla Protein Powder, which is vegan and doesn't contain any artificial sweeteners.

Per serving: Calories: 350; Fat: 11g; Protein: 19g; Carbohydrates: 50g; Fiber: 11g; Sugar: 29g

Aloha Banana Toast

Prep time: 5 minutes / Serves 1

QUICK

NO COOK

5-INGREDIENT

1 slice sprouted grain or whole wheat toast

1 tablespoon natural almond butter

1 banana, sliced

1 tablespoon unsweetened coconut flakes

1 teaspoon chia seeds

Dash ground cinnamon

1. After toasting the bread to desired level of doneness, spread the almond butter on it. Top it with the banana slices.

2. Sprinkle on the coconut flakes, chia seeds, and cinnamon.

 Smart shopping: After years of enjoying gourmet toasts, I have found that the crunchier and crispier the toast is, the better the end result will be. I like Dave's Killer Bread for this reason; it's nice and seedy.

Per serving: Calories: 374; Fat: 15g; Protein: 11g; Carbohydrates: 55g; Fiber: 12g; Sugar: 21g

Power Muesli

Prep time: 5 minutes, plus overnight to chill / Serves 4

2 cups old fashioned (or gluten-free) oats

½ cup chopped dates

¼ cup chopped cashews

3 tablespoons chia seeds

½ teaspoon ground cinnamon

3½ cups nondairy milk of choice

½ cup blackberries

1. In a bowl, mix together the oats, dates, cashews, chia seeds, and cinnamon.

2. Add the milk and stir until combined.

3. Transfer the mixture into 4 mason jars or other containers with airtight lids. Refrigerate the muesli overnight; it will soften as it sits.

4. Remove the muesli from the refrigerator, top it with blackberries, and eat it cold.

 Make ahead: This is a great meal to prep for the week. It will stay fresh in the refrigerator for up to five days.

Per serving: Calories: 332; Fat: 12g; Protein: 10g; Carbohydrates: 50g; Fiber: 11g; Sugar: 14g

Chia Pudding, Three Ways

Prep Time: 5 minutes, plus 4 hours to chill / Serves 2

SOY-FREE

GLUTEN-FREE

For the pudding base

1 cup unsweetened
   almond milk

¼ cup chia seeds

Vanilla

½ cup plain Coconut
   Yogurt (page 146)

2 tablespoons
   maple syrup

1 teaspoon gluten-free
   vanilla extract

Pinch salt

PB and Chocolate

2 tablespoons
   cocoa powder

1 teaspoon gluten-free
   vanilla extract

2 tablespoons chunky
   natural peanut butter

1 tablespoon
   chopped dates

Tropical Pineapple

5 tablespoons (2 scoops)
   vanilla protein powder

½ cup diced
   fresh pineapple

2 teaspoons maple syrup

1 teaspoon
   coconut extract

1. In a medium bowl, combine the almond milk and chia seeds. Add the ingredients from the flavor of your choice, omitting any optional toppings.

2. Divide the mixture between 2 (8-ounce) mason jars or airtight containers, seal, and refrigerate for at least 4 hours.

3. When you're ready to eat, stir the pudding well and add any optional toppings.

Smart shopping: I recommend IdealRaw Vanilla Protein Powder, which is vegan and doesn't contain any artificial sweeteners. If you don't want to make your own coconut yogurt, I recommend the brands So Delicious, Silk, or Coconut Dream.

Variation tip: I don't usually recommend toppings, since it's easy to overload on sugar. But if you need a big breakfast to recover from a workout or get you through the day, go for it. For the vanilla, I recommend topping with berries, hemp seeds, and a dash of cinnamon. For the peanut butter and chocolate, try dark chocolate shavings and chopped peanuts. For the tropical pineapple, toasted coconut and more fresh pineapple is a winning combination.

Per serving (Vanilla): Calories: 356; Fat: 22g; Protein: 6g; Carbohydrates: 50g; Fiber: 9g; Sugar: 15g

Per serving (Peanut Butter and Chocolate): Calories: 274; Fat: 17g; Protein: 9g; Carbohydrates: 21g; Fiber: 13g; Sugar: 4g

Per serving (Tropical Pineapple): Calories: 302; Fat: 13g; Protein: 20g; Carbohydrates: 25g; Fiber: 12g; Sugar: 10g

Quick Apple-Cinnamon Oatmeal

Prep time: 5 minutes / Cook time: 5 minutes / Serves 3

SOY-FREE

QUICK

ONE POT

GLUTEN-FREE OPTION

5-INGREDIENT

1½ cups old fashioned (or gluten-free) oats

1 apple, unpeeled and diced

1 teaspoon ground cinnamon

3 tablespoons almond butter

Liquid stevia (optional)

1. In a medium saucepan over high heat, bring 3 cups of water to a boil.

2. Lower the heat to medium, add the oats and apples, and cook, stirring frequently, for 4 to 5 minutes, until all the moisture is gone. Remove from the heat.

3. Add the cinnamon and almond butter and stir to combine. Sweeten to taste with liquid stevia (if using).

4. Divide the mixture equally between 3 bowls and serve, or store the mixture in an airtight container in the refrigerator for up to 4 days.

 Ingredient tip: Oatmeal is a great source of fiber. Eat it one hour before you work out to avoid exercising on an empty stomach or try some after you exercise to recover from all the exertion.

Per serving: Calories: 280; Fat: 12g; Protein: 9g; Carbohydrates: 39g; Fiber: 8g; Sugar: 8g

Carrot Cake Oatmeal

Prep time: 10 minutes / Cook time: 5 minutes / Serves 3

1½ cups unsweetened almond milk

1½ teaspoons ground cinnamon

½ teaspoon ground ginger

½ teaspoon ground nutmeg

½ teaspoon ground cloves

Pinch salt

¾ cup grated carrots

¾ cup old fashioned oats

1 tablespoon vanilla extract

5 drops liquid stevia (optional)

2 tablespoons almond butter

5 tablespoons (2 scoops) vanilla protein powder

3 teaspoons slivered almonds

1. In a small saucepan over medium heat, mix together the milk, cinnamon, ginger, nutmeg, cloves, salt, and ½ cup of water.

2. Stir in the carrots and oats, bring to a gentle simmer, and cook for 3 to 4 minutes, stirring frequently, until the liquid evaporates. Remove from the heat.

3. Add the vanilla, stevia (if using), almond butter, and protein powder and stir to combine.

4. Divide the mixture equally between 3 bowls and top each with the almonds, or store the mixture in an airtight container in the refrigerator for up to 4 days.

 Cooking tip: If your oatmeal is too thick, add 1 additional tablespoon of almond milk.

 Smart shopping: I recommend IdealRaw Vanilla Protein Powder, which is vegan and doesn't contain any artificial sweeteners.

Per serving: Calories: 281; Fat: 13g; Protein: 16g; Carbohydrates: 24g; Fiber: 6g; Sugar: 4g

French Toast, Two Ways

Prep time: 5 minutes / Cook time: 5 minutes / Serves 4

SOY-FREE

QUICK

1 cup Homemade Almond Milk (page 145)

2 tablespoons cashew butter

1 tablespoon ground flaxseeds

⅛ teaspoon salt

1 tablespoon olive oil

4 slices thick, whole grain bread

For a sweet version

1 tablespoon coconut sugar

½ teaspoon vanilla extract

Sweet toppings: 1 cup fresh berries of choice

For a savory version

⅓ cup chickpea flour

2 tablespoons nutritional yeast

Savory toppings: ¼ sliced avocado, 1 teaspoon chives, dash hot sauce

1. In a high-powered blender, combine the almond milk, cashew butter, flaxseeds, and salt. Add the ingredients for the sweet or savory version (except for the toppings) and blend on high for about 1 minute, until smooth.

2. Place the batter in a wide, shallow bowl and dredge each slice of bread in the mixture, making sure to coat both sides.

3. In a large skillet over medium-high heat, warm the olive oil. Add the bread slices and cook for about 2 minutes on each side, until browned.

4. Place each slice of French toast on its own plate and top with the sweet or savory version's toppings as desired.

Per Serving (Sweet, 1 slice): Calories: 127; Fat: 8g; Protein: 3g; Carbohydrates: 13g; Fiber: 2g; Sugar: 8g

Per serving (Savory, 1 slice): Calories: 290; Fat: 15g; Protein: 11g; Carbohydrates: 32g; Fiber: 8g; Sugar: 7g

Triple Berry Coconut Parfait

Prep time: 10 minutes / Cook time: 25 minutes / Serves 4

Nonstick cooking spray

1 cup old fashioned (or gluten-free) oats

½ cup chopped cashews

2 tablespoons chia seeds

2 tablespoons ground flaxseeds

½ teaspoon salt

½ teaspoon ground cinnamon

½ cup chopped pitted dates

2 cups Coconut Yogurt (page 146)

2 cups berries of your choice

1. Preheat the oven to 350°F. Line a baking sheet with aluminum foil and spray it with nonstick cooking spray.

2. In a medium bowl, mix together the oats, cashews, chia seeds, flaxseeds, salt, and cinnamon. Set aside.

3. In a food processor or high-powered blender, combine the dates and ½ cup of water and pulse until a paste forms.

4. Add the paste to the oat mixture and stir to combine. Spread the mixture evenly onto the prepared baking sheet.

5. Bake for 12 minutes. Flip the mixture carefully and continue baking for an additional 12 minutes. Let the mixture cool completely on a wire rack.

6. Divide the yogurt between 4 bowls. Top each bowl with ¼ cup of the oat mixture and ½ cup of the berries. Serve immediately.

 Smart shopping: If you don't want to make your own coconut yogurt, I recommend the brands So Delicious, Silk, or Coconut Dream.

Per serving: Calories: 612; Fat: 40g; Protein: 11g; Carbohydrates: 50g; Fiber: 9g; Sugar: 22g

Everything Bagel Sweet Potatoes

Prep time: 5 minutes / Cook time: 20 minutes / Serves 8

ONE POT

NUT-FREE

GLUTEN-FREE

5-INGREDIENT

2 large sweet potatoes, cut lengthwise into ¼-inch slices

Coconut oil cooking spray

½ teaspoon sea salt

16 tablespoons vegan cream cheese

16 thick slices hothouse tomatoes

8 teaspoons Everything Bagel Seasoning (page 140) or store-bought

5 tablespoons plus 1 teaspoon chives

1. Preheat the oven to 400°F. Place a wire rack on top of a baking sheet or line the baking sheet with parchment paper.

2. Place the sweet potatoes on the prepared baking sheet. Spray them with a small amount of cooking spray and sprinkle them with sea salt.

3. Roast for 20 minutes. Let them cool on a wire rack for 10 minutes.

4. Spread each sweet potato slice with 1 tablespoon of vegan cream cheese. Top each with a tomato slice, ½ teaspoon of the bagel seasoning, and 1 teaspoon of the chives.

5. Serve immediately, or store them in an airtight container in the refrigerator for up to 7 days. To reheat, place them in a toaster oven until warmed through.

 Smart shopping: For the vegan cream cheese, I recommend buying Tofutti brand. Whatever brand you buy, be sure to look for a non-hydrogenated version!

Per serving (2 slices): Calories: 122; Fat: 5g; Protein: 2g; Carbohydrates: 14g; Fiber: 2g; Sugar: 4g

Roasted Sweet Potato Hash

Prep time: 10 minutes / Cook time: 35 minutes / Serves 4

Nonstick cooking spray

2 large sweet
potatoes, diced

1 red or green bell
pepper, diced

1 tablespoon olive oil

1 teaspoon paprika

1 teaspoon dried thyme

½ teaspoon dried parsley

¼ teaspoon salt

1. Preheat the oven to 450°F. Line a baking sheet
   with aluminum foil and spray with nonstick
   cooking spray.

2. In a medium bowl, toss the sweet potatoes and
   bell pepper with the oil. Add the paprika, thyme,
   parsley, and salt and toss again to coat.

3. Spread the potatoes out on the prepared baking
   sheet. Bake for 30 to 35 minutes, or until the
   potatoes are tender.

GLUTEN-FREE

5-INGREDIENT

Per serving: Calories: 128; Fat: 4g; Protein: 2g; Carbohydrates: 23g; Fiber: 4g; Sugar: 6g

Southwest Scrambled "Eggs"

Prep time: 10 minutes / Cook time: 15 minutes / Serves 4

QUICK

ONE POT

NUT-FREE

GLUTEN-FREE

1 tablespoon olive oil

¼ cup diced yellow onion

2 garlic cloves, minced

1 (14-ounce) package extra-firm lite tofu, pressed and drained overnight

1 cup diced red bell pepper

1 (15-ounce) can black beans, drained and rinsed

2 teaspoons chili powder

1 teaspoon ground cumin

1 teaspoon dried oregano

½ teaspoon ground turmeric

1. In a large nonstick skillet over medium heat, warm the olive oil.

2. Add the onion and garlic and cook for about 2 minutes. Crumble the tofu into the skillet, stir to combine, and cook for about 5 minutes, until lightly browned. Do not stir.

3. Add the red bell pepper, black beans, chili powder, cumin, oregano, and turmeric and stir to combine. Cook for another 5 minutes, until heated through. Serve hot.

Ingredient tip: Tofu is best prepared after as much liquid as possible has been removed from it. To do this, place a block of tofu between two clean dish towels, place a heavy object (such as a book) on top of the towel, and let it sit overnight. This will result in the perfect texture for cooking.

Per serving: Calories: 265; Fat: 10g; Protein: 18g; Carbohydrates: 28g; Fiber: 11g; Sugar: 3g

Spring Vegetable Muffins

Prep time: 15 minutes / Cook time: 35 minutes / Makes 12 muffins

Nonstick cooking spray

1½ cups chickpea flour

¼ cup nutritional yeast

1 teaspoon baking powder

1 teaspoon garlic salt

1 teaspoon dried basil

¾ cup chopped
asparagus spears

¾ cup chopped red
bell pepper

¼ cup chopped red onion

½ cup chopped
fresh spinach

1. Preheat the oven to 350°F. Lightly grease a 12-cup muffin tin with nonstick cooking spray and set aside.

2. In a medium bowl, combine the chickpea flour, yeast, baking powder, garlic salt, and basil. Add 2¼ cups of water and stir until combined.

3. Add the asparagus, bell pepper, onion, and spinach and stir to combine.

4. Spoon ¼ cup of the batter into each muffin tin.

5. Bake for 35 minutes, or until browned and a toothpick inserted into the center of a muffin comes out clean. Let the muffins cool completely on a wire rack. The muffins will firm up as they cool.

 Love your leftovers: These will keep in the refrigerator for about four to five days, or in the freezer for up to two months.

Per serving (2 muffins): Calories: 122; Fat: 2g; Protein: 9g; Carbohydrates: 18g; Fiber: 5g; Sugar: 4g

SOY-FREE

NUT-FREE

GLUTEN-FREE

Chipotle Breakfast Burrito

Prep time: 15 minutes / Cook time: 35 minutes / Serves 8

For the sweet potato hash

Nonstick cooking spray

2 large sweet potatoes, diced

1 green bell pepper, diced

1 tablespoon olive oil

1 teaspoon paprika

1 teaspoon dried thyme

½ teaspoon dried parsley

¼ teaspoon salt

For the tofu "eggs"

1 tablespoon olive oil

1 (14-ounce) package extra-firm lite tofu, pressed and drained overnight

2 tablespoons nutritional yeast

For the chipotle sauce

½ cup Coconut Yogurt (page 146)

1 chipotle in adobo sauce

1 garlic clove

1 tablespoon lime juice

⅛ teaspoon ground cumin

To make the sweet potato hash

1. Preheat the oven to 450°F. Line a baking sheet with aluminum foil and spray with nonstick cooking spray.

2. In a medium bowl, toss the sweet potato and bell pepper with the oil. Add the paprika, thyme, parsley, and salt and toss again to coat.

3. Place the seasoned potatoes on the prepared baking sheet. Bake for 30 to 35 minutes, or until potatoes are tender. Set aside.

To make the tofu "eggs"

4. While the sweet potatoes are roasting: In a medium skillet over medium-high heat, warm the oil. Crumble the tofu into the pan, sprinkle with the yeast, and stir to combine. Cook for about 5 minutes, until the yeast is completely absorbed. Set aside.

To make the sauce

5. In a high-powered blender, combine the yogurt, chipotle, garlic, lime juice, and cumin and blend on high for about 1 minute, until smooth.

For the burritos

4 whole wheat or low-carb wraps

1 (15-ounce) can black beans, drained and rinsed

1 cup salsa

To assemble the burritos

6. Place the whole wheat wraps on a clean work surface. Add ¼ of the tofu, beans, salsa, and sweet potato mixture in the center of each wrap. Top each with 1 tablespoon of the sauce. Fold the sides of the wrap inward, and then roll up until the ingredients are tucked inside.

7. Cut each burrito in half and enjoy.

Ingredient tip: Tofu is best prepared after as much liquid as possible has been removed from it. To do this, place a block of tofu between two clean dish towels, place a heavy object (such as a book) on top of the towel, and let it sit overnight. This will result in the perfect texture for cooking.

Love your leftovers: Wrap leftover burritos tightly in plastic wrap, then place them in a freezer-safe storage bag, making sure to squeeze out all the air before sealing. The burritos can be stored in the refrigerator for up to three days or in the freezer for up to one month.

Smart shopping: I like Cut Da Carb wraps, which are vegan, low-carb, and hold up to this hearty burrito.

Per serving: Calories: 284; Fat: 10g; Protein: 13g; Carbohydrates: 35g; Fiber: 10g; Sugar: 5g

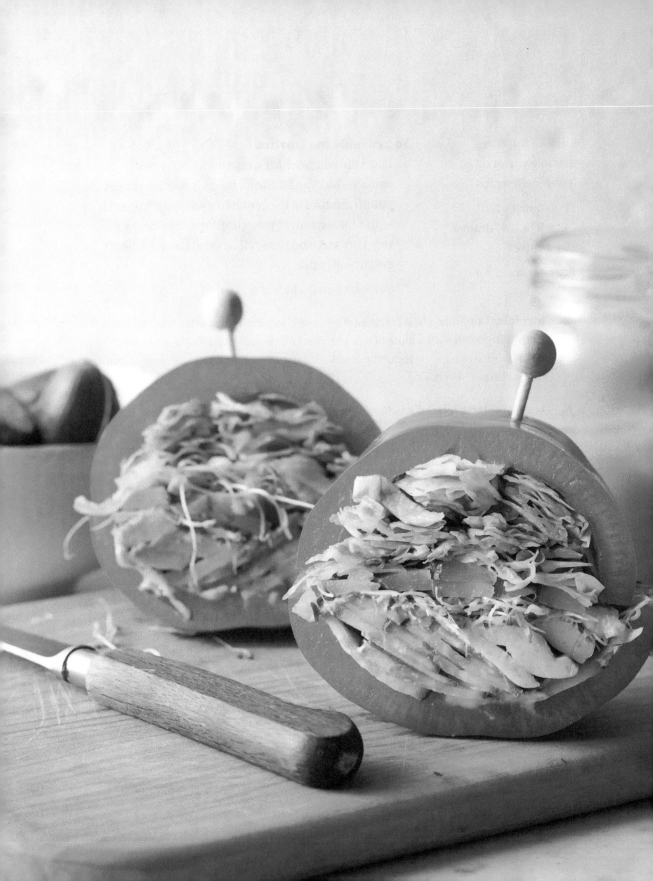

CHAPTER 4

Salads and Handhelds

< Loaded Bell Pepper Sandwich, page 69

Pomegranate-Cabbage Salad

Prep time: 5 minutes / Cook time: 5 minutes / Serves 1

QUICK

ONE POT

GLUTEN-FREE

5-INGREDIENT

Nonstick cooking spray

2 cups shredded cabbage

½ cup chopped
    extra-firm lite tofu,
    pressed and drained

2 tablespoons liquid
    coconut aminos

⅓ cup pomegranate seeds

2 tablespoons
    slivered almonds

1. Spray a medium nonstick pan with nonstick
   cooking spray and set it over medium heat. Add the
   cabbage and cook for 3 to 4 minutes, until soft.

2. Add the tofu and cook, stirring frequently for 1 to
   2 minutes, until warm.

3. Remove the pan from the heat and stir in the
   coconut aminos.

4. Top the salad with the pomegranate seeds and
   slivered almonds. Serve warm.

 Cooking tip: Don't be intimidated by how much cabbage this recipe requires. It will cook
down and end up at about half the amount you started with.

 Swap it: You can use low-sodium soy sauce instead of the coconut aminos.

Per serving: Calories: 290; Fat: 14g; Protein: 17g; Carbohydrates: 32g; Fiber: 8g;
Sugar: 21g

Edamame and Snow Pea Power Salad

Prep time: 10 minutes / Cook time: 10 minutes / Serves 4

QUICK

ONE POT

NUT-FREE

GLUTEN-FREE

For the salad

½ cup multicolored quinoa, rinsed

1 pound frozen shelled edamame, thawed

1 pound snow peas, cut diagonally into ⅛-inch slices

6 radishes, thinly sliced

For the dressing

4 tablespoons rice wine vinegar

2 tablespoons olive oil

5 to 6 drops liquid stevia

2 teaspoons toasted sesame oil

2 teaspoons soy sauce

2 tablespoons sesame seeds

To make the salad

1. In a medium saucepan over high heat, mix together the quinoa and 1 cup of water and bring to a boil. Reduce the heat to low and simmer for about 10 minutes, until the quinoa has absorbed all the liquid. Fluff the quinoa with a fork and set aside.

2. While the quinoa is cooking: In a large microwavable bowl, combine the edamame and ¼ cup of water. Microwave on high for 4 to 6 minutes, until bright green and crisp-tender. Drain and set aside to cool.

3. In a large bowl, mix together the quinoa, edamame, snow peas, and radishes. Set aside.

To make the dressing

4. In a small bowl, whisk together the vinegar, olive oil, stevia, sesame oil, and soy sauce. Add the dressing to the vegetables and quinoa and stir to combine.

5. Divide the salad between 4 bowls and sprinkle each one with sesame seeds.

 Swap it: If snow peas don't appeal to you, feel free to add in any raw vegetable you like. Some of my favorites are zucchini, cucumber, and broccoli.

Per serving (2 cups): Calories: 389; Fat: 18g; Protein: 23g; Carbohydrates: 37g; Fiber: 10g; Sugar: 8g

Kale Caesar Salad

Prep time: 20 minutes / Serves 2

SOY-FREE

QUICK

5-INGREDIENT

1 large bunch kale, ribs removed, torn into bite-size pieces

1 cup of Lemon Tahini Dressing (page 141)

1½ cups Roasted Chickpeas (page 106)

1. Place the kale in a large bowl.

2. Pour the dressing over the kale and toss to coat. Refrigerate for 10 to 15 minutes.

3. Add the chickpeas to the kale, toss well, and serve.

 Cooking tip: Refrigerating the salad gives the dressing some time to tenderize the kale.

 Love your leftovers: If you're saving half of this salad for later, store half the chickpeas separately.

Per serving: Calories: 357; Fat: 21g; Protein: 13g; Carbohydrates: 33g; Fiber: 12g; Sugar: 6g

Meatless Taco Salad

Prep time: 10 minutes / Cook time: 10 minutes / Serves 1

Nonstick cooking spray

½ cup Easy Lentils
(page 121)

2 tablespoons Taco
Seasoning (page 138)
or store-bought

2 cups romaine lettuce

¼ cup cooked black
beans, drained
and rinsed

¼ cup corn

¼ cup diced
cherry tomatoes

2 tablespoons Not-So-
Spicy Jalapeño Hummus
(page 144)

2 tablespoons salsa

1. Spray a large skillet with nonstick cooking spray
   and set it over medium heat. Add the lentils and
   cook for 5 minutes.

2. Add the taco seasoning and ¼ cup of water and stir
   to combine. Lower the heat to medium-low and
   simmer, stirring occasionally, for about 5 minutes,
   until the liquid is mostly gone. Set aside to cool.

3. To assemble the salad: Place the lettuce in a bowl
   and top it with the lentils, black beans, corn, and
   cherry tomatoes. Spoon the hummus and salsa on
   top and give it a quick stir to combine.

SOY-FREE

QUICK

NUT-FREE

GLUTEN-FREE

Ingredient tip: Most store-bought taco seasonings contain MSG, so I highly recommend using my Taco Seasoning instead. It will last for up to three months in your pantry, and you'll use it all the time.

Love your leftovers: This salad can be stored in an airtight container in the refrigerator for up to three days.

Per serving: Calories: 384; Fat: 9g; Protein: 20g; Carbohydrates: 62g; Fiber: 18g; Sugar: 11g

Baked Falafel Salad

Prep time: 20 minutes, plus 30 minutes to chill / Cook time: 30 minutes / Serves 4

SOY-FREE

NUT-FREE

GLUTEN-FREE

For the falafel

1½ cups canned chickpeas, drained and rinsed

1 cup chopped cilantro

1 cup chopped Italian parsley

3 garlic cloves

½ cup roughly chopped red onion

2 tablespoons freshly squeezed lime juice

1 teaspoon freshly ground black pepper

1 teaspoon sea salt

1 teaspoon ground cumin

1 teaspoon dried basil

1 teaspoon dried oregano

¼ cup chickpea flour

Nonstick cooking spray

To make the falafel

1. In a food processor, combine the chickpeas, cilantro, parsley, garlic, onion, lime juice, pepper, salt, cumin, basil, and oregano. Pulse until the mixture forms a paste.

2. Add the chickpea flour and pulse, scraping down the sides of the food processor frequently, until fully combined.

3. Transfer the falafel mixture to a small bowl, cover, and refrigerate for 30 minutes to set.

4. Preheat the oven to 375°F. Line a baking sheet with aluminum foil and spray with nonstick cooking spray.

5. Form the falafel mixture into 12 tablespoon-size balls and place them on the prepared baking sheet.

6. Spray the back of a small spatula with nonstick cooking spray and gently press down on each falafel to make flattened disks.

7. Bake for 30 minutes, or until the falafel are cooked through. Let cool completely before serving.

8. The falafel can be stored in an airtight container in the refrigerator for up to 6 days.

For one serving of salad

2 cups mixed greens

½ avocado, sliced

½ cup sliced cucumber

¼ lemon, sliced

2 tablespoons Lemon
Tahini Dressing
(page 141)

½ teaspoon dried parsley

To make the salad

9. Be sure to multiply the salad ingredients based on how many servings you need. Place the mixed greens in a large salad bowl. Arrange the sliced avocado, cucumber, and lemon on top of the greens.

10. Place 3 falafel on top of the salad and drizzle it with the dressing. Sprinkle it with parsley and serve immediately.

Per serving: Calories: 166; Fat: 6g; Protein: 7g; Carbohydrates: 24g; Fiber: 8g; Sugar: 5g

Toasted Lavash and Chickpea Salad

Prep time: 30 minutes / Cook time: 35 minutes / Serves 4

For the pita chips

2 sheets Joseph's Lavash Bread

Nonstick cooking spray

Sea salt

For the chickpeas

1 (15-ounce) can chickpeas, drained and rinsed

1 tablespoon olive oil

½ teaspoon ground cumin

½ teaspoon ground chili powder

½ teaspoon salt

For the dressing

4 tablespoons olive oil

Juice of 1 lemon

1½ tablespoons red wine vinegar

1 teaspoon Dijon mustard

1 teaspoon dried oregano

5 to 6 drops liquid stevia

To make the pita chips

1. Preheat the oven to 400°F. Line a baking sheet with aluminum foil and have another unlined baking sheet ready.

2. Cut the lavash bread in half, lengthwise, into 2 long rectangles, and then cut them into smaller bite-size triangles. Place the triangles on the unlined baking sheet, spray them with nonstick cooking spray, and sprinkle them with sea salt.

3. Bake for 5 minutes, flip the triangles over, and bake for another 3 minutes, or until crunchy. Set aside to cool.

To make the chickpeas

4. In a small bowl, mix together the chickpeas, olive oil, cumin, chili powder, and salt. Spread the chickpea mixture evenly onto the prepared baking sheet.

5. Bake for 12 minutes. Toss the mixture and bake for another 12 minutes, or until golden brown.

To make the dressing

6. In a small bowl, whisk together the olive oil, lemon juice, vinegar, mustard, oregano, and stevia.

For the salad

2 cups cooked
Israeli couscous

1 medium
cucumber, chopped

1 cup halved
cherry tomatoes

¼ cup chopped
fresh parsley

½ cup chopped roasted
red bell pepper

To make the salad

7. In a large bowl, mix together the couscous,
cucumber, tomatoes, parsley, and roasted
bell pepper.

8. Pour the dressing over the salad and mix well.

9. Spoon the chickpeas over the salad, arrange the
toasted lavash around the edges, and serve.

 Smart shopping: I like to use Joseph's Lavash Bread. If you have trouble finding lavash bread, use a Flatout protein wrap or a whole wheat pita.

Per serving: Calories: 419; Fat: 21g; Protein: 14g; Carbohydrates: 47g; Fiber: 10g; Sugar: 6g

Spinach and Avocado Pasta Salad

Prep time: 10 minutes / Cook time: 15 minutes / Serves 6

SOY-FREE

QUICK

NUT-FREE

For the pasta

1 (16-ounce) package
farfalle pasta

2 cups diced
cherry tomatoes

½ red onion, diced

4 cups chopped
fresh spinach

1 avocado, diced

For the dressing

3 garlic cloves, minced

3 tablespoons olive oil

1 teaspoon salt

1 teaspoon freshly ground
black pepper

To make the pasta

1. In a large pot of water over high heat, cook the pasta according to the package instructions. Drain, rinse with cold water, and set aside.

2. In a medium bowl, mix together the tomatoes and onion.

3. Add the pasta to the tomato mixture and stir gently. Add the spinach and avocado and mix together.

To make the dressing

4. In a small bowl, whisk together the garlic, olive oil, salt, and pepper.

To assemble the salad

5. Add the dressing to the pasta and toss until everything is coated. Serve immediately.

 Cooking tip: This salad is best made right before serving. Assemble the ingredients at the last minute for the freshest (and most delicious) salad possible.

Per serving (2 cups): Calories: 407; Fat: 12g; Protein: 12g; Carbohydrates: 64g; Fiber: 5g; Sugar: 5g

Loaded Bell Pepper Sandwich

Prep time: 10 minutes / Serves 1

1 red bell pepper, halved
  lengthwise and seeded

½ cup torn
  iceberg lettuce

1 tablespoon
  Dijon mustard

½ cup sliced cucumber

½ avocado, sliced

½ large hothouse
  tomato, sliced

2 pickle spears, halved
  lengthwise if needed

⅓ cup alfalfa sprouts

1. Place the pepper halves, cut-side up, on a plate.
2. Fill one pepper half with the lettuce.
3. Spread the mustard on the other pepper half.
4. Add the cucumber, avocado, tomato, pickles, and sprouts. Press the two pepper halves back together to form a sandwich and cut it in half. Use toothpicks to hold it together until ready to eat.

Variation tip: This might seem like an unconventional way to make a sandwich, but give it a go and you will be hooked! Feel free to experiment with any other vegetables you have on hand. Leftover roasted veggies, pickled cabbage, or even some dairy-free cheese slices could work well, too.

Per serving: Calories: 199; Fat: 12g; Protein: 5g; Carbohydrates: 22g; Fiber: 11g; Sugar: 10g

The Best Black Bean Burgers

Prep time: 25 minutes, plus 30 minutes to chill / Cook time: 15 minutes / Serves 10

SOY-FREE

NUT-FREE

2 slices toasted whole wheat bread

2 tablespoons olive oil, divided

1 medium onion, chopped

2 garlic cloves, minced

2 tablespoons minced jalapeño pepper

1 teaspoon ground cumin

1 (15-ounce) can black beans, drained and rinsed

1¼ cups cooked brown rice

1 teaspoon freshly squeezed lime juice

½ teaspoon salt

½ teaspoon freshly ground black pepper

¼ cup chopped fresh cilantro

6 Bibb lettuce leaves

1 medium cucumber, sliced

1 medium tomato, sliced

1. Line a baking sheet with parchment paper.

2. Rip the bread slices in pieces and put them into a food processor. Pulse until the bread forms crumbs. Transfer the crumbs to a bowl and set aside.

3. In a large skillet over medium heat, warm 1 tablespoon of olive oil. Add the onion, garlic, jalapeño, and cumin. Cook, stirring, for 2 minutes.

4. Transfer the onion mixture to the food processor. Add the black beans, brown rice, lime juice, salt, and pepper. Pulse until the beans are chopped but not pureed. Transfer the mixture to a large bowl, add half of the bread crumbs and the cilantro, and stir until combined. If the mixture is sticky, add more bread crumbs. Any leftover bread crumbs can be stored in a zip-top bag in the freezer for up to 4 months.

5. Using your hands, form the mixture into 10 patties and place them on the prepared baking sheet. Cover the patties with plastic wrap and refrigerate for at least 30 minutes, or until firm.

6. In a large skillet over high heat, warm the remaining 1 tablespoon of olive oil. Add the patties to the pan and cook for 4 to 5 minutes on each side, until browned. Transfer the cooked patties to paper towels and let them cool for a bit. You may need to cook the patties in batches.

7. Right before serving, place each burger in a lettuce cup and top with slices of cucumber and tomato.

Ingredient tip: These taste great with a dollop of my Not-So-Spicy Jalapeño Hummus (page 144) or a good Dijon mustard.

Love your leftovers: The recipe makes 10 patties, so prior to cooking them, freeze any you won't be eating right away in a single layer in a gallon- or quart-size zip-top bag for up to four months. Thaw in the refrigerator overnight before cooking.

Per serving (1 patty): Calories: 134; Fat: 4g; Protein: 5g; Carbohydrates: 22g; Fiber: 5g; Sugar: 3g

Ultimate Veggie Sandwich

Prep time: 20 minutes / Serves 1

QUICK

NUT-FREE

NO COOK

3 tablespoons Not-So-Spicy Jalapeño Hummus (page 144)

2 slices toasted Ezekiel bread or other whole wheat bread

⅓ cup chopped fresh spinach leaves

½ Roma tomato, sliced

½ avocado, sliced

¼ cup sliced red onion

¼ cup julienned carrots

½ cucumber, cut into ribbons with a vegetable peeler

⅓ cup alfalfa sprouts

1 dill pickle, halved

Spread half the hummus on each slice of bread. Place the spinach on one of the bread slices. Add layers of the tomato, avocado, onion, carrots, cucumber, sprouts, and pickles. Top with the second slice of bread, hummus-side down, and enjoy.

Technique tip: To cut julienned vegetables: First, peel the vegetable. Cut the veggie horizontally into ⅛-inch sections. Stack the slices on top of one another and cut long slices as thin as possible. This will leave you with perfect matchstick-size pieces.

Variation tip: Divide the ingredients between the two slices of bread and serve them as an open-faced sandwich.

Per serving: Calories: 485; Fat: 23g; Protein: 19g; Carbohydrates: 61g; Fiber: 18g; Sugar: 9g

Pesto and Tomato Panini

Prep time: 5 minutes / Cook time: 10 minutes / Serves 1

For the pesto

1½ cups packed fresh
basil leaves

2 garlic cloves

⅓ cup cashews

⅓ cup olive oil

½ teaspoon salt

For the sandwich

Nonstick cooking spray

2 slices sourdough bread

1 tablespoon olive oil

⅓ cup vegan mozzarella
shreds (optional)

5 thin slices Roma tomato

¼ cup basil leaves, torn
into small pieces

½ cup spinach, torn into
small pieces

Freshly ground
black pepper

To make the pesto

1. Combine the basil, garlic, cashews, olive oil, and
salt in a food processor and pulse until creamy.

To make the sandwich

2. Place a small skillet over medium–high heat and
spray well with nonstick cooking spray.

3. Brush 1 side of each slice of bread with the olive oil.
Spread ½ tablespoon of pesto on the other side of
each bread slice.

4. Place one slice of bread, oil-side down, in the
skillet. Add the vegan mozzarella (if using), tomato,
basil, and spinach. Season with pepper.

5. Top with the other slice of bread, oil-side up, and
cook for about 4 minutes, until the bread is golden.

6. Carefully flip the sandwich and cook for another
2 to 3 minutes, until golden brown.

7. Cut the sandwich in half and serve.

 Appliance tip: If you have a panini press, cook the sandwich for about four minutes total. Cut it in half before serving.

 Love your leftovers: The pesto can be stored in an airtight container in the refrigerator for up to seven days or in the freezer for up to two months.

 Smart shopping: I like Daiya brand "mozzarella" shreds.

Per serving: Calories: 667; Fat: 35g; Protein: 17g; Carbohydrates: 75g; Fiber: 5g; Sugar: 9g

Easy Mediterranean Quesadilla

Prep time: 5 minutes / Cook time: 20 minutes / Serves 1

SOY-FREE

QUICK

ONE POT

NUT-FREE

5-INGREDIENT

Nonstick cooking spray

1 cup chopped spinach

½ cup black beans

1 (8-inch) flour tortilla

¼ cup Not-So-Spicy Jalapeño Hummus (page 144)

⅓ cup sliced kalamata olives

1. Spray a medium skillet with nonstick cooking spray and set it over medium-high heat. Add the spinach and cook, stirring, for about 3 minutes, until wilted. Once it's wilted, place the spinach on a plate and set aside.

2. Spray the pan with nonstick cooking spray again. Add the black beans and cook, stirring, for about 3 minutes, until heated through. Transfer the cooked beans to a bowl and set aside. Carefully wipe out the pan.

3. Heat the tortilla in the pan over medium heat for about 1 minute on each side. Spread the hummus on half of the tortilla and add the spinach, black beans, and olives. Fold the tortilla in half and continue to cook for 3 to 4 minutes on each side, until golden brown. Let cool for about 2 minutes.

4. Cut the quesadilla into triangles and enjoy it warm.

Per serving: Calories: 604; Fat: 35g; Protein: 18g; Carbohydrates: 59g; Fiber: 13g; Sugar: 2g

Chickpea Salad Pinwheels

Prep time: 15 minutes / Serves 4

1 (15-ounce) can chickpeas, drained and rinsed

⅓ cup finely chopped celery

¼ cup finely chopped radishes

½ teaspoon salt

½ teaspoon freshly ground black pepper

½ teaspoon garlic powder

¼ teaspoon paprika

3 tablespoons Vegan Mayo (page 136)

3 tablespoons Dijon mustard

4 (8-inch) whole grain tortillas

2 cups torn fresh spinach

1. In a small bowl, mash the chickpeas with a fork until they are broken up well, but before they form a paste.

2. Add the celery, radishes, salt, pepper, garlic powder, and paprika and mix until combined. Add the vegan mayo and mustard, stir to combine, and set aside.

3. To assemble the wrap: Lay the tortillas on a clean work surface. Place ½ cup of the spinach in a vertical line down the center of one tortilla. Add ½ cup of the chickpea mixture over the spinach and spread it evenly. Repeat with the remaining tortillas.

4. Roll the tortillas up tightly. Cut each tortilla crosswise into 1-inch pinwheels and serve.

Variation tip: This can easily be made into a sandwich by using two slices of Ezekiel bread (a sprouted-grain bread found in the freezer section of most grocery stores) or another whole wheat bread.

Per serving (1 wrap): Calories: 274; Fat: 6g; Protein: 12g; Carbohydrates: 44g; Fiber: 6g; Sugar: 3g

Spring Vegetable Rolls with Peanut Sauce

Prep time: 15 minutes / Serves 1

QUICK

NO COOK

GLUTEN-FREE

For the peanut sauce

1 tablespoon peanut butter powder

1 garlic clove, minced

½ tablespoon minced ginger

1 tablespoon tamari (for gluten-free option) or low-sodium soy sauce

Liquid stevia

For the spring rolls

2 rice paper sheets or 1 low-carb tortilla

½ cup julienned cucumber

¼ cup shredded carrots

2 large slices of avocado

2 cilantro sprigs

½ cup extra-firm lite tofu, pressed and drained overnight

To make the peanut sauce

1. In a small bowl, mix together the peanut butter powder, garlic, ginger, tamari, stevia to taste, and 2 tablespoons of water. Set aside.

To make the spring rolls

2. Carefully dip the rice paper sheets into warm water to soften them. Set aside. If you are using the tortilla, cut it in half to make 2 rolls.

3. Lay 1 rice paper sheet on a plate and place half of the cucumber, carrots, avocado, cilantro, and tofu in the center. Fold in the sides, and then roll it up like a burrito. Repeat with the second rice paper sheet. Serve with the sauce on the side for dipping.

Ingredient tip: Tofu is best prepared after as much liquid as possible has been removed from it. To do this, place a block of tofu between two clean dish towels, place a heavy object (such as a book) on top of the towel, and let it sit overnight. This will result in the perfect texture for cooking.

Smart shopping: Peanut butter powder is a fairly new product that can be found at most major grocery stores in the baking aisle or by the peanut butter. My favorite brand is Better Body Foods, but PB2 is another great and fairly common brand.

Technique tip: To cut julienned vegetables: First, peel the vegetable. Cut the veggie horizontally into ⅛-inch sections. Stack the slices on top of one another and cut long slices as thin as possible. This will leave you with perfect matchstick-size pieces.

Per serving (2 spring rolls): Calories: 255; Fat: 9g; Protein: 17g; Carbohydrates: 31g; Fiber: 6g; Sugar: 4g

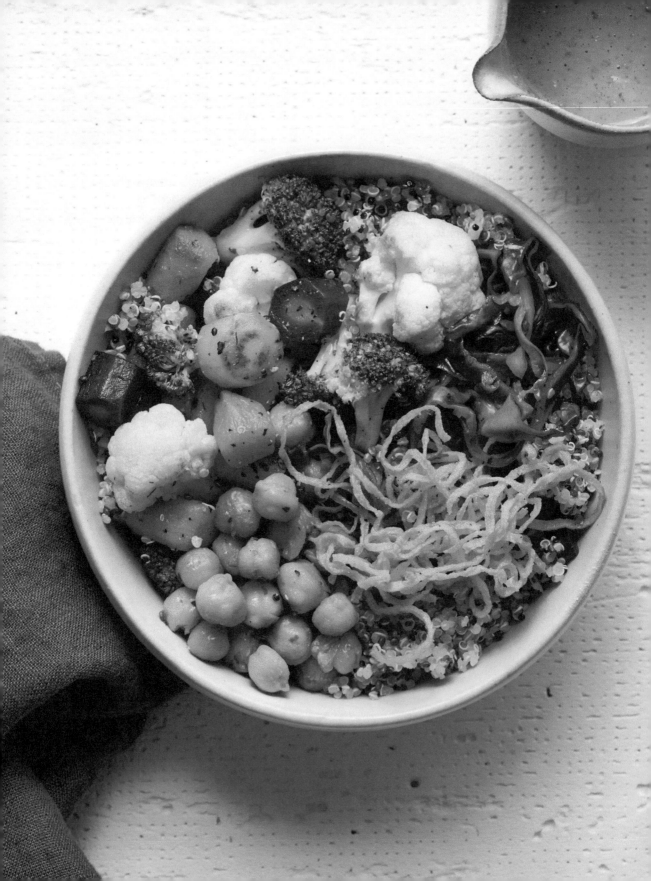

Mains

< Green Goddess Buddha Bowl, page 90

Superfood Pesto Zoodles

Prep time: 10 minutes / Cook time: 10 minutes / Serves 2

SOY-FREE

QUICK

GLUTEN-FREE

For the pesto

1½ cups packed
   fresh basil

2 garlic cloves

⅓ cup cashews

⅓ cup olive oil

½ teaspoon salt

For the zoodles

2 medium
   zucchini, spiralized

⅛ cup pesto

1 cup halved
   cherry tomatoes

1 cup shelled frozen
   edamame, thawed

½ cup Vegan Parmesan
   (page 135)

To make the pesto

1. In a food processor, combine the basil, garlic, cashews, olive oil, and salt and process until creamy.

To make the zoodles

2. In a large nonstick skillet over medium heat, cook the zucchini noodles for 1 to 2 minutes, until softened.

3. Add the pesto and tomatoes and stir to combine. Cover and continue to cook for another 3 to 4 minutes, until heated through.

4. Add the edamame and vegan Parmesan and stir to combine. Serve immediately.

 Love your leftovers: Store any leftover pesto in a small glass jar with an airtight lid. You can use it as a spread on sandwiches, a sauce for pasta, and even on top of some avocado toast. It will stay fresh for about five days in the refrigerator or up to two months in the freezer.

Per serving (1 cup): Calories: 525; Fat: 34g; Protein: 29g; Carbohydrates: 34g; Fiber: 15g; Sugar: 11g

Pumpkin-Sage Pasta

Prep time: 10 minutes / Cook time: 15 minutes / Serves 6

1 (8-ounce) box penne chickpea pasta

1 cup pumpkin puree

1 cup raw cashews, soaked in water for at least 1 hour and drained

1 cup unsweetened almond milk

1 tablespoon lemon juice

3 garlic cloves, minced

½ teaspoon salt

¼ teaspoon ground nutmeg

2 tablespoons chopped fresh sage

1. Cook the pasta in a large stockpot according to the package instructions. Drain and return the pasta to the pot.

2. Combine the pumpkin puree, cashews, almond milk, lemon juice, garlic, salt, and nutmeg in a food processor and pulse until smooth.

3. Pour the sauce over the pasta and stir until well coated.

4. Spoon the pasta into bowls and top each with fresh sage.

 Smart shopping: For the chickpea pasta, I recommend Banza. If you're having trouble finding that brand, you can also use another legume-based pasta, such as red lentil pasta.

Per serving: Calories: 292; Fat: 12g; Protein: 15g; Carbohydrates: 35g; Fiber: 7g; Sugar: 4g

Perfect Mac and Cheese

Prep time: 5 minutes / Cook time: 15 minutes / Serves 2

SOY-FREE

QUICK

ONE POT

¾ cup cashew milk

3 tablespoons
nutritional yeast

2 tablespoons
arrowroot powder

½ teaspoon salt

½ teaspoon
onion powder

½ teaspoon garlic powder

½ teaspoon
ground mustard

3 cups cooked pasta
shells, zoodles, or
cauliflower rice

1. In a small saucepan over medium heat, combine the cashew milk, yeast, arrowroot powder, salt, onion powder, garlic powder, and mustard and cook, whisking, until it begins to boil.

2. Lower the heat to medium and continue whisking for about 1 more minute, until the sauce thickens.

3. Place the pasta in a large bowl. Pour the sauce over the shells, stir to combine, and serve.

 Smart shopping: Banza, Explore Cuisine, and Tolerant Organic are all healthy pasta brands that can be found in most major grocery stores. Premade zucchini noodles or riced cauliflower can also often be found in the prepared-foods area of the produce section.

Per serving (1½ cups): Calories: 338; Fat: 3g; Protein: 16g; Carbohydrates: 62g; Fiber: 6g; Sugar: 1g

Pad Thai

Prep time: 10 minutes / Cook time: 15 minutes / Serves 4

1 (8-ounce) package
   brown rice noodles

½ cup chopped cilantro

½ cup tamari (for
   gluten-free option) or
   low-sodium soy sauce

⅓ cup smooth
   peanut butter

1 garlic clove, minced

Juice of 1 lime

2 tablespoons olive oil

Nonstick cooking spray

3 cups shredded carrots

3 cups snap peas

½ cup minced scallions

4 tablespoons
   sesame seeds

QUICK

GLUTEN-FREE

1. Cook the pasta according to the package instructions. Drain the pasta and set aside.

2. While the pasta is cooking: In a small bowl, whisk together the cilantro, tamari, peanut butter, garlic, lime juice, and olive oil. Set aside.

3. Spray a large pot with nonstick cooking spray and set it over medium-high heat. Add the carrots and snap peas and cook, stirring, for 6 to 8 minutes. Add the noodles and peanut butter mixture and cook, stirring, for another 2 to 3 minutes, until heated through. Remove from the heat.

4. Divide the noodle mixture between 4 bowls, sprinkle each with 2 tablespoons of scallions and 1 tablespoon of sesame seeds, and serve.

 Smart shopping: Most conventional peanut butter brands contain hydrogenated oil. When choosing a more natural option, make sure the peanut butter has the least amount of ingredients possible. If you see just peanuts and salt on the label, you know you've found the right brand.

Per serving: Calories: 531; Fat: 24g; Protein: 17g; Total Carbs: 66g; Fiber: 11g; Sugar: 9g

Spaghetti and "Meatballs"

Prep time: 20 minutes / Cook time: 30 minutes / Makes 24 "meatballs"

For the "meatballs"

3 tablespoons olive
   oil, divided

3 garlic cloves

⅓ cup panko
   bread crumbs

2 tablespoons
   ground flaxseed

⅓ cup chopped
   sun-dried tomatoes

⅓ cup minced fresh basil

⅓ cup nutritional yeast

Pinch red pepper flakes

¼ teaspoon salt

⅛ teaspoon freshly
   ground black pepper

1 (16-ounce) can
   chickpeas, drained
   and rinsed

To make the "meatballs"

1. Preheat the oven to 375°F.

2. In a large skillet over medium heat, warm
   1 tablespoon of olive oil. Add the garlic and cook for
   2 minutes. Place the garlic in a food processor or
   blender. Set the skillet aside.

3. Add the bread crumbs, flaxseed, sun-dried
   tomatoes, basil, yeast, red pepper, salt, pepper, and
   1 tablespoon of olive oil to the food processor or
   blender with the garlic and pulse until well blended.

4. Add the chickpeas to the food processor or blender
   and pulse until a stiff dough forms. If the dough is
   too dry to stick together, add a little water and pulse
   a few times.

5. Using a tablespoon, form the dough into
   24 "meatballs."

6. Return the skillet to the stove and warm the
   remaining 1 tablespoon of olive oil over high heat.
   Add the "meatballs" and cook, turning them
   frequently, for 4 to 5 minutes, until browned.

7. Place the "meatballs" on a baking sheet and bake
   for 15 minutes. Set aside.

For the marinara sauce

1 (28-ounce) can San Marzano tomatoes

2 tablespoons olive oil

2 garlic cloves, minced

½ teaspoon dried oregano

½ teaspoon dried basil

½ teaspoon salt

2 teaspoons coconut sugar, plus more as needed (optional)

Roasted Spaghetti Squash (page 130)

To make the marinara sauce

8. Using your hands, crush the tomatoes into a large bowl. Set aside.

9. In a large saucepan over medium-high heat, warm the olive oil. Add the garlic and cook for about 1 minute. Add the oregano, basil, and salt and cook for another 2 minutes.

10. Lower the heat to medium, add the tomatoes, stir to combine, and simmer for about 20 minutes, until the liquid reduces.

11. Taste the sauce and if it seems acidic, add 2 teaspoons of coconut sugar (if using) and stir to combine. Taste the sauce again and add more coconut sugar if needed.

To serve

12. Place the spaghetti squash on plates and top it with the sauce and "meatballs."

 Smart shopping: If you don't want to make your own marinara sauce, look for a low-sugar natural brand like Rao's or Newman's Own Organic. Similarly, if you don't want to roast your own spaghetti squash, you can often find a precooked version in the produce section of your local grocery store.

 Love your leftovers: The marinara sauce can be stored in an airtight container in the refrigerator for up to five days or in the freezer for up to two months.

Per serving (3 "meatballs," 1½ cups spaghetti squash, ½ cup marinara): Calories: 237; Fat: 14g; Protein: 7g; Carbohydrates: 23g; Fiber: 6g; Sugar: 7g

Easy Marinara Lentils

Prep time: 10 minutes / Cook time: 25 minutes / Serves 2

For the marinara sauce

1 (28-ounce) can San Marzano tomatoes

2 tablespoons olive oil

2 garlic cloves, minced

½ teaspoon dried oregano

½ teaspoon dried basil

½ teaspoon salt

2 teaspoons coconut sugar, plus more if needed (optional)

For the lentils and broccoli

1 cup lentils

6 cups chopped broccoli

1 cup marinara sauce

4 tablespoons Vegan Parmesan (page 135)

To make the marinara sauce

1. Using your hands, crush the tomatoes into a large bowl. Set aside.

2. In a large saucepan over medium-high heat, warm the olive oil. Add the garlic and cook for about 1 minute. Add the oregano, basil, and salt and cook for another 2 minutes.

3. Reduce the heat to medium, add the tomatoes, stir to combine, and simmer for about 20 minutes, until the liquid reduces.

4. Taste the sauce and if it seems acidic, add 2 teaspoons coconut sugar (if using) and stir to combine. Taste the sauce again and add more coconut sugar if needed.

To make the lentils and broccoli

5. In a small saucepan over high heat, bring 1½ cups of water to a boil. Add the lentils and stir to combine. Reduce the heat to low, cover, and simmer for about 20 minutes, until tender. Remove from the heat and set aside.

6. While the lentils are cooking: Pour 1 inch of water into a saucepan big enough to hold a steamer basket. Bring the water to a boil over medium-high heat. Put the broccoli inside the steamer basket and place the basket into the saucepan. Cover and steam for 4 to 8 minutes, until the broccoli is cooked to your liking.

7. To serve, divide the lentils between two bowls. Top each bowl with half the broccoli and ½ cup of the marinara sauce. Sprinkle the vegan Parmesan over the top.

Love your leftovers: The marinara sauce can be stored in an airtight container in the refrigerator for up to five days or in the freezer for up to two months.

Technique tip: If you don't have a steamer basket, you can easily steam the broccoli in the microwave. Place the florets in a microwave-safe bowl with about 2 tablespoons of water and cover it with a paper towel. Microwave on high for about four minutes, then carefully remove it.

Per serving: Calories: 630; Fat: 15g; Protein: 40g; Carbohydrates: 95g; Fiber: 24g; Sugar: 14g

Cashew and Tofu Stir-Fry

Prep time: 5 minutes / Cook time: 5 minutes / Serves 1

QUICK

ONE POT

GLUTEN-FREE

Nonstick cooking spray

1 cup frozen
cauliflower rice

1 cup frozen
stir-fry vegetables

1 cup chopped kale leaves

3 tablespoons tamari (for
gluten-free option) or
low-sodium soy sauce

½ cup extra-firm
lite tofu, pressed
and drained
overnight, cubed

1 tablespoon
chopped cashews

1. Spray a medium skillet with nonstick cooking spray
   and set it over medium heat. Add the cauliflower
   rice, stir-fry vegetables, and kale and cook for 2 to
   3 minutes, until crisp-tender.

2. Add the tamari and tofu, stir to combine, and cook
   for about 1 minute.

3. Transfer the mixture to a plate. Sprinkle it with the
   cashews and serve.

Per serving: Calories: 220; Fat: 7g; Protein: 21g; Carbohydrates: 20g; Fiber: 6g; Sugar: 7g

Tofu and Rainbow Veggies

Prep time: 15 minutes / Cook time: 15 minutes / Serves 6

Nonstick cooking spray

1 (14-ounce) package
extra-firm lite tofu,
pressed and drained
overnight, cubed

2 cups diced
broccoli florets

2 cups quartered
mushrooms

2 cups cubed
butternut squash

1 zucchini, cut into
1-inch pieces

1 yellow squash, cut into
1-inch pieces

1 red bell pepper, cut into
1-inch pieces

1 onion, cut into
1-inch pieces

2 tablespoons olive oil

4 tablespoons
balsamic vinegar

4 garlic cloves, peeled

4 tablespoons
fresh thyme

1 tablespoon salt

1 teaspoon freshly ground
black pepper

1. Preheat the oven to 425°F. Line a large baking sheet
   with aluminum foil and spray it with nonstick
   cooking spray.

2. Place the tofu, broccoli, mushrooms, butternut
   squash, zucchini, yellow squash, bell pepper,
   and onion on the prepared baking sheet and toss
   with the olive oil, vinegar, garlic, thyme, salt, and
   pepper. Spread the tofu and vegetables out in a
   single layer.

3. Roast for 12 to 15 minutes, until tender and
   slightly browned.

4. Serve this dish hot or store it in an airtight
   container in the refrigerator for up to 3 days.

QUICK

NUT-FREE

GLUTEN-FREE

Per serving: Calories: 173; Fat: 7g; Protein: 10g; Total Carbs: 21g; Fiber: 6g; Sugar: 7g

Green Goddess Buddha Bowl

Prep time: 35 minutes / Cook time: 25 minutes / Serves 2

For the roasted vegetables

4 cups chopped vegetables such as broccoli, cauliflower, or rainbow carrots

2 tablespoons olive oil

½ teaspoon salt

½ teaspoon freshly ground black pepper

For the sweet potato spirals

1 cup coconut oil

1 medium sweet potato, spiralized

1 teaspoon sea salt

To roast the vegetables

1. Preheat the oven to 425°F. Line a baking sheet with aluminum foil.

2. On the prepared baking sheet, toss the vegetables with the olive oil. Add the salt and pepper and toss again. Arrange the vegetables in a single layer.

3. Roast for 25 minutes. Set aside.

To make the sweet potato spirals

4. In a medium skillet over low heat, warm the coconut oil. Increase the heat slowly to medium-high until the oil is slightly bubbling.

5. Add the sweet potato spirals and salt to the pan and fry for 8 to 10 minutes, until the spirals shrink in size and are slightly browned.

6. Place the spirals on a paper towel to drain.

For each salad

2 cups greens of choice

⅓ cup cooked quinoa

1 cup roasted vegetables

⅓ cup Roasted Chickpeas
(page 106)

½ cup sliced purple
cabbage, raw or pickled

Half of the sweet
potato spirals

2 tablespoons Green
Goddess Dressing
(page 142)

To assemble the salad

7. Place the greens in a large bowl. Add the quinoa, roasted vegetables, chickpeas, cabbage, and sweet potato spirals.

8. Add the dressing, toss to combine, and serve.

 Love your leftovers: This salad will last up to four days in the refrigerator. Store the dressing and sweet potato spirals in individual containers. You can eat this salad cold, but I like to warm up the quinoa, roasted vegetables, and sweet potato spirals in the microwave for 30 to 45 seconds first.

Per serving: Calories: 678; Fat: 58g; Protein: 11g; Carbohydrates: 33g; Fiber: 9g; Sugar: 6g

Tex-Mex Enchilada Bake

Prep time: 10 minutes / Cook time: 45 minutes / Serves 6

SOY-FREE

NUT-FREE

GLUTEN-FREE

Nonstick cooking spray

1 cup quinoa

2 cups Vegetable
Broth (page 134)
or store-bought

1 tablespoon olive oil

½ cup chopped
white onion

1 red bell pepper, diced

2 garlic cloves, minced

1 (15-ounce) can
low-sodium enchilada
sauce (check label
for gluten-free
and soy-free)

2 (15-ounce) cans
black beans, drained
and rinsed

1 (15.25-ounce) can corn,
drained and rinsed

1 teaspoon salt

¼ cup chopped
fresh cilantro

1. Preheat the oven to 350°F. Spray a 9-by-13-inch baking dish with nonstick cooking spray and set aside.

2. In a medium saucepan over high heat, combine the quinoa and broth and bring to a boil. Reduce the heat to low, cover, and cook for about 15 minutes, until the liquid is absorbed. Remove from the heat and fluff with a fork.

3. While the quinoa is cooking: In a small pan over medium-high heat, warm the olive oil. Add the onion, bell pepper, and garlic and cook, stirring constantly, for 5 minutes. Remove from the heat, add the enchilada sauce, black beans, corn, and salt, and mix well.

4. Transfer the vegetable mixture and quinoa to the baking dish, stir to combine, and spread it evenly in the dish.

5. Bake for 20 minutes. Let it cool briefly on a wire rack. Sprinkle the cilantro over the top and serve.

 Love your leftovers: This will keep in the refrigerator for up to five days or up to four weeks in the freezer.

Per serving: Calories: 346; Fat: 7g; Protein: 14g; Carbohydrates: 58g; Fiber: 14g; Sugar: 7g

Vegan Shepherd's Pie

Prep time: 15 minutes / Cook time: 40 minutes / Serves 6

SOY-FREE

NUT-FREE

GLUTEN-FREE

For the mashed potatoes

3 pounds russet potatoes, peeled and diced

4 tablespoons olive oil

1 teaspoon salt

½ teaspoon freshly ground black pepper

For the filling

Nonstick cooking spray

1 medium white onion, diced

2 garlic cloves, minced

1½ cups red lentils

4 cups Vegetable Broth (page 134) or store-bought

1 teaspoon dried thyme

1 (12-ounce) package frozen vegetable medley (peas, carrots, green beans, and corn)

To make the mashed potatoes

1. Place the potatoes in a large stockpot over medium-high heat and cover them with water. Bring it to a boil, reduce the heat to medium, and simmer gently for about 30 minutes, until tender. Drain the water and keep the potatoes in the pot.

2. Add the olive oil, salt, and pepper and mash with a potato masher or hand mixer until no lumps remain. Set aside.

To make the filling

3. Preheat the oven to 450°F. Spray a 9-by-13-inch baking dish with nonstick cooking spray. Set aside.

4. Spray a medium skillet with nonstick cooking spray and set it over medium-high heat. Add the onion and garlic and cook for about 3 minutes, until fragrant. Add the lentils, broth, and thyme; stir and bring to a boil.

5. Reduce the heat to medium-low and simmer for about 20 minutes, until the lentils are tender.

6. Add the frozen vegetables and cook, stirring, for another 10 minutes. Remove from the heat.

7. Spoon the lentil mixture into the baking dish and spread it out evenly. Top with the mashed potatoes. Bake for 10 to 15 minutes, or until the potatoes are slightly browned.

8. Let cool for about 15 minutes before serving.

 Love your leftovers: Store any leftovers in the refrigerator for up to four days.

Per serving: Calories: 519; Fat: 14g; Protein: 19g; Carbohydrates: 84g; Fiber: 11g; Sugar: 3g

Cauliflower Tacos

Prep time: 10 minutes / Cook time: 25 minutes / Serves 4

SOY-FREE

NUT-FREE

GLUTEN-FREE

1 large head cauliflower, cut into bite-size pieces

2 tablespoons olive oil

1 teaspoon chili powder

½ teaspoon onion powder

½ teaspoon ground cumin

½ teaspoon salt

½ teaspoon freshly ground black pepper

1 (14-ounce) package coleslaw

Lemon Tahini Dressing (page 141)

1 avocado, chopped

8 corn tortillas

1. Preheat the oven to 425°F. Line a baking sheet with aluminum foil and set it aside.

2. In a large mixing bowl, mix together the cauliflower, olive oil, chili powder, onion powder, cumin, salt, and pepper.

3. Spread the mixture evenly on the prepared baking sheet and bake for 25 minutes, flipping the cauliflower with a spatula halfway through.

4. While the cauliflower is cooking: In a medium bowl, toss the coleslaw with the dressing, cover, and refrigerate it until ready to use.

5. To assemble the tacos: Divide the coleslaw, roasted cauliflower, and chopped avocado between the tortillas and serve.

Variation tip: Try these tacos with my Not-So-Spicy Jalapeño Hummus (page 144) for a different flavor profile.

Per serving (2 tacos): Calories: 427; Fat: 26g; Protein: 12g; Carbohydrates: 46g; Fiber: 14g; Sugar: 9g

Lemon Pepper Tofu Steak with Broccoli

Prep time: 10 minutes / Cook time: 25 minutes / Serves 6

Nonstick cooking spray

½ cup panko
  bread crumbs

2 garlic cloves, minced

1 tablespoon chopped
  fresh parsley

1 tablespoon chopped
  fresh basil

Zest of 1 lemon, grated

½ teaspoon salt, divided

¼ teaspoon freshly
  ground black pepper

1 tablespoon olive oil

1 (14-ounce) package
  extra-firm lite tofu,
  pressed and drained

1 broccoli head, cut
  into florets

Juice of 1 lemon

Lemon wedges,
  for garnish

1. Preheat the oven to 400°F. Line a baking sheet with aluminum foil and spray it with nonstick cooking spray.

2. In a small bowl, mix together the bread crumbs, garlic, parsley, basil, lemon zest, ¼ teaspoon of salt, and pepper. Add the olive oil and mix well.

3. Pat the tofu completely dry with paper towels and cut it into 6 (½-inch-thick) slices. Place the tofu slices in one layer on the prepared baking sheet and spoon the bread crumb mixture over each "steak." Press the mixture gently with the back of a spoon.

4. Bake for 25 minutes.

5. While the tofu is baking: Place the broccoli and 2 tablespoons of water in a microwave-safe bowl, cover it with plastic wrap, and microwave on high for 4 minutes. Drain, sprinkle the broccoli with the remaining ¼ teaspoon of salt, and mix well.

6. Top each tofu steak with a squeeze of lemon juice and fresh lemon wedges, and serve warm with the broccoli.

Per serving: Calories: 130; Fat: 4g; Protein: 10g; Carbohydrates: 15g; Fiber: 4g; Sugar: 2g

Slow Cooker Sweet Potato Curry

Prep time: 20 minutes / Cook time: 8 hours / Serves 8

1 (13.5-ounce) can light coconut milk

2 cups pumpkin puree

2 cups Vegetable Broth (page 134) or store-bought

2 teaspoons Garam Masala (page 139) or store-bought

1½ teaspoons curry powder

1 teaspoon salt

¼ teaspoon freshly ground black pepper

¼ teaspoon ground turmeric

½ onion, diced

2 garlic cloves, minced

3 carrots, chopped

3 cups cubed sweet potato

2 (16-ounce) cans chickpeas, drained and rinsed

½ cup raw cashews

Juice of 1 lime

1. In a slow cooker, combine the coconut milk, pumpkin puree, vegetable broth, garam masala, curry powder, salt, pepper, and turmeric and whisk well until blended.

2. Add the onion, garlic, carrots, sweet potato, chickpeas, cashews, and lime juice and stir to combine.

3. Cook on low for 6 to 8 hours, until the vegetables are tender enough to pierce with a fork.

4. Serve hot. This curry tastes delicious on its own or over rice, quinoa, or zucchini noodles.

Love your leftovers: This makes a big batch of curry, which can be stored in the freezer for up to two months. Seal the leftovers in a gallon-size freezer bag (a quart-size bag can work, as well, for smaller portions) and place the bag directly on a freezer shelf. This will help the curry freeze flat so it can be stacked for efficient storage. Thaw it in the refrigerator overnight before reheating it.

Stovetop instructions: In a large stockpot over medium-high heat, combine the coconut milk, pumpkin puree, and vegetable broth and whisk until smooth. Add the garam masala, curry, salt, pepper, turmeric, onion, garlic, carrots, and sweet potato, stir to combine, and bring the mixture to a boil. Reduce the heat to medium-low and simmer for about 20 minutes, until the vegetables are tender. Add the chickpeas and remove the pot from the heat. Squeeze in the lime juice, stir in the cashews, and serve.

Per serving (1 cup): Calories: 307; Fat: 10g; Protein: 9g; Carbohydrates: 48g; Fiber: 10g; Sugar: 12g

Thai-Inspired Coconut Curry

Prep time: 10 minutes / Cook time: 20 minutes / Makes 6 cups

SOY-FREE

QUICK

ONE POT

GLUTEN-FREE

1 tablespoon coconut oil

1 onion, diced

1 red bell pepper, diced

8 Yukon Gold potatoes, scrubbed and diced

3 cups chopped broccoli

1 cup Vegetable Broth (page 134) or store-bought

1 (13.5-ounce) can light coconut milk

1 (14-ounce) can fire-roasted tomatoes

4 tablespoons red curry paste

4 garlic cloves, minced

1-inch piece of fresh ginger, minced

2 cups grated carrots

3 cups fresh spinach

1 lime, halved

3 cups riced cauliflower

1. In a large stockpot over medium heat, warm the coconut oil. Add the onion and cook, stirring occasionally, for 4 minutes.

2. Add the bell pepper, potatoes, and broccoli and cook, stirring occasionally, for 5 minutes.

3. Add the vegetable broth, coconut milk, roasted tomatoes, curry paste, garlic, and ginger, stir, and bring the mixture to a boil. Add the carrots and simmer for 5 to 7 minutes, until the carrots are tender.

4. Add the spinach, stir to combine, and cook for 1 minute.

5. Squeeze in the lime juice and stir. Serve over riced cauliflower.

Per serving (2 cups): Calories: 306; Fat: 8g; Protein: 9g; Carbohydrates: 56g; Fiber: 10g; Sugar: 11g

Corn Chowder

Prep time: 15 minutes / Cook time: 25 minutes / Serves 6

Nonstick cooking spray

1 onion, chopped

3 garlic cloves, minced

4 large russet potatoes,
  peeled and diced

3 carrots, peeled
  and diced

4 cups Vegetable
  Broth (page 134)
  or store-bought

2 cups frozen corn

½ teaspoon dried thyme

1 tablespoon chopped
  fresh parsley

1 teaspoon salt

1 bay leaf

2 tablespoons
  nutritional yeast

1 cup unsweetened
  almond milk

3 tablespoons arrowroot
  powder (optional)

½ cup chopped scallions,
  for topping

1. Spray a large stockpot with nonstick cooking spray and set it over medium-high heat. Add the onion and garlic and cook, stirring, for about 2 minutes, until fragrant.

2. Add the potatoes and carrots and cook, stirring, for another 5 minutes.

3. Add the broth, corn, thyme, parsley, salt, and bay leaf, cover, and bring to a boil. Reduce the heat to medium and simmer, covered, for about 15 minutes, until the carrots are tender.

4. Discard the bay leaf. Using an immersion blender, pulse the soup mixture for 1 to 2 minutes, until it begins to thicken. If you don't own an immersion blender, you can transfer the mixture to a regular blender instead and blend it for one minute on low.

5. Add the yeast, almond milk, and arrowroot powder (if using) and whisk until everything is blended. Top with the scallions and serve warm.

SOY-FREE ONE POT GLUTEN-FREE

Ingredient tip: Arrowroot powder is a grain-free alternative to flour and is used to thicken sauces and soups.

Per serving (1½ cups): Calories: 331; Fat: 4g; Protein: 9g; Total Carbs: 68g; Fiber: 7g; Sugar: 7g

Black Bean and Sweet Potato Tortilla Soup

Prep time: 10 minutes / Cook time: 25 minutes / Serves 6

SOY-FREE

ONE POT

NUT-FREE

GLUTEN-FREE

½ cup quinoa

½ tablespoon olive oil

4 garlic cloves, minced

2 cups diced onion

½ teaspoon salt

¼ teaspoon freshly ground black pepper

1 large sweet potato, scrubbed and diced

2 teaspoons ground cumin

½ teaspoon chili powder

½ teaspoon ground coriander

6 cups Vegetable Broth (page 134) or store-bought

1 (15-ounce) can black beans, drained and rinsed

⅓ cup blue corn tortilla chips

1. Cook the quinoa according to package instructions. Set aside.

2. In a large pot over medium-high heat, warm the olive oil. Add the garlic and onion and cook for 5 minutes. Add the salt, pepper, and sweet potato and cook for an additional 5 minutes.

3. Stir in the cumin, chili powder, coriander, and broth and bring it to a boil. Reduce the heat to medium and simmer for about 15 minutes, until the vegetables are tender.

4. Add the black beans and quinoa right before serving. Spoon the soup into bowls and top them with tortilla chips.

 Smart shopping: For the tortilla chips, I like the brand Garden of Eatin' because they're gluten-free and don't use genetically modified organisms (non-GMO).

Per serving (1 cup): Calories: 274; Fat: 8g; Protein: 9g; Carbohydrates: 43g; Fiber: 10g; Sugar: 7g

Coconut-Lime Noodle Soup

Prep time: 10 minutes / Cook time: 20 minutes / Serves 4

1 tablespoon olive oil

2 teaspoons red
curry paste

2 teaspoons
lemongrass paste

4 cups Vegetable
Broth (page 134)
or store-bought

1 cup sliced red
bell pepper

1 cup chopped asparagus

½ cup sliced carrots

1 (13.5-ounce) can light
coconut milk

2 (7-ounce) packages
shirataki noodles

½ cup sliced mushrooms

1 lime, halved

4 teaspoons sesame seeds

Fresh cilantro,
for garnish

1. In a large stockpot over medium-high heat, warm the olive oil. Add the red curry paste and lemongrass paste and cook, stirring constantly, for 3 minutes.

2. Add the broth, bell pepper, asparagus, and carrots and bring it to a boil. Reduce the heat to medium-low and simmer for about 10 minutes, until the asparagus is bright green.

3. Add the coconut milk, noodles, and mushrooms and simmer for an additional 5 minutes.

4. Squeeze in the lime juice and remove the pot from the heat. Spoon the soup into bowls and top each one with 1 teaspoon of sesame seeds and a few sprigs of fresh cilantro.

SOY-FREE

QUICK

ONE POT

GLUTEN-FREE

Ingredient tip: Shirataki noodles are Japanese noodles made with Asian yams. They're a great low-calorie, carb-free swap for regular noodles. You can find them at the grocery store in the pasta or international goods section, or you can order them online. Most packages contain two servings, but check the serving size before using two packages in this recipe.

Per serving: Calories: 194; Fat: 16g; Protein: 3g; Carbohydrates: 14g; Fiber: 6g; Sugar: 5g

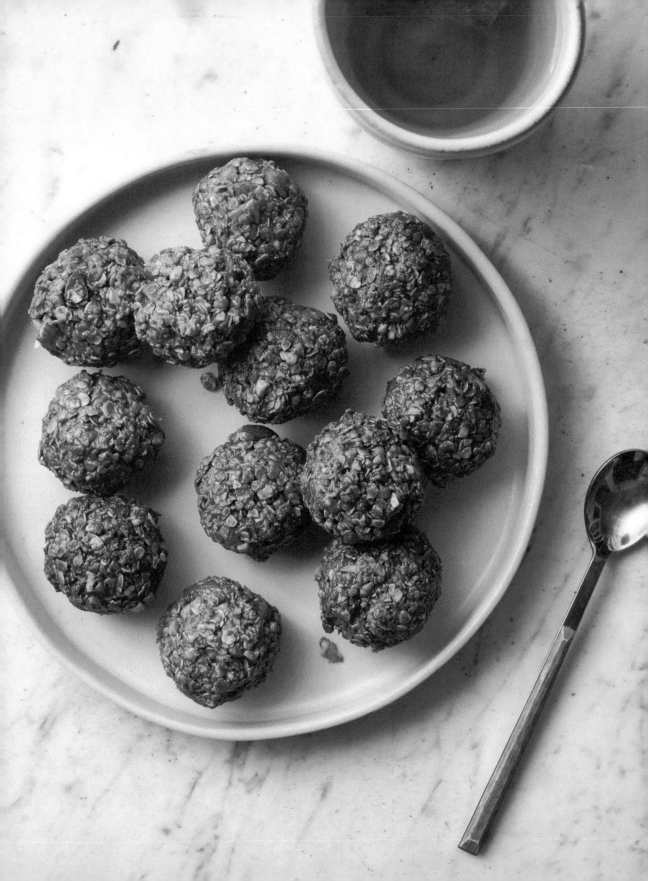

CHAPTER 6

Snacks and Treats

< **Coconut Brownie Truffles, page 109**

Kale Chips

Prep time: 10 minutes / Cook time: 20 minutes / Serves 4

SOY-FREE

QUICK

ONE POT

NUT-FREE

GLUTEN-FREE

5-INGREDIENT

6 ounces curly kale, stemmed and torn into pieces

2 tablespoons olive oil

1/3 cup nutritional yeast

2 teaspoons onion powder

1 teaspoon salt

1 teaspoon garlic powder

1/2 teaspoon cayenne pepper

1. Preheat the oven to 325°F. Line a baking sheet with aluminum foil and set aside.

2. Wash the kale thoroughly and spin it in a salad spinner or pat dry. Make sure the leaves are completely dry before moving to step 3.

3. In a medium bowl, toss the kale with the olive oil. Massage the kale with your hands for 3 to 4 minutes, or until each piece of kale is completely coated with oil. Set aside.

4. In a small bowl, combine the yeast, onion powder, salt, garlic powder, and cayenne pepper.

5. Add the seasoning to the kale and toss until completely combined. Spread the kale in a single layer on the prepared baking sheet. Bake for 10 minutes, rotate the pan, and bake for another 10 minutes.

6. Let the kale chips cool completely. They will crisp up as they cool.

 Love your leftovers: Kale chips are best stored in a zip-top bag at room temperature for up to three days.

Per serving (1 cup): Calories: 108; Fat: 7g; Protein: 6g; Carbohydrates: 6g; Fiber: 3g; Sugar: 1g

Crispy Garlic Edamame

Prep time: 10 minutes / Cook time: 20 minutes / Serves 6

12 ounces frozen shelled edamame, thawed

1 tablespoon avocado oil

1 teaspoon garlic salt

1 teaspoon minced garlic

1. Preheat the oven to 425°F. Line a baking sheet with parchment paper and set it aside.

2. Pat dry the edamame with a paper towel. In a small bowl, mix together the edamame, avocado oil, garlic salt, and minced garlic.

3. Spread the edamame in a single layer on the prepared baking sheet.

4. Roast for 16 minutes, shaking the pan halfway through.

5. Allow the edamame to cool slightly and serve warm or at room temperature.

 Cooking tip: The drier the edamame, the easier the oil and spices will stick to it, resulting in better flavor. So, after thawing, make sure to dry the soybeans really well.

Per serving (⅓ cup): Calories: 97; Fat: 5g; Protein: 8g; Carbohydrates: 7g; Fiber: 2g; Sugar: 1g

QUICK

NUT-FREE

GLUTEN-FREE

5-INGREDIENT

Roasted Chickpeas, Four Ways

Prep time: 5 minutes / Cook time: 30 minutes / Serves 14

SOY-FREE

ONE POT

NUT-FREE OPTION

GLUTEN-FREE

5-INGREDIENT

For the chickpea base

2 (15-ounce) cans
chickpeas, drained
and rinsed

2 tablespoons olive oil

Curry-Spice

2 teaspoons curry powder

1 teaspoon chili powder

1 teaspoon Garam Masala
(page 139)

½ teaspoon salt

Cinnamon Sugar

2 teaspoons
ground cinnamon

4 tablespoons
coconut sugar

½ teaspoon salt

Barbecue Roasted

1 teaspoon
smoked paprika

1 teaspoon
cayenne pepper

1 teaspoon onion powder

½ teaspoon garlic salt

Salty and Spicy

½ teaspoon red
pepper flakes

1 teaspoon sea salt

1. Preheat the oven to 350°F. Line a baking sheet with aluminum foil or parchment paper.

2. Spread the chickpeas over a clean kitchen towel and press them gently with paper towels to dry thoroughly.

3. Transfer the chickpeas to a medium bowl, drizzle them with the olive oil, and toss to coat.

4. In a small bowl, combine the ingredients of your choice of flavorings. Add them to the chickpeas and toss to coat.

5. Spread out the chickpeas on the prepared baking sheet and roast for 15 minutes. Stir the chickpeas and roast for an additional 15 minutes. Repeat as many times as necessary until the chickpeas are crispy and brown.

6. Let the chickpeas cool before serving.

Love your leftovers: The roasted chickpeas can be stored in an airtight container or a zip-top bag at room temperature for up to three days.

Smart shopping: Don't want to make your own Garam Masala? Find it in the spices aisle of the grocery store.

Per serving (Curry-Spice, ¼ cup): Calories: 72; Fat: 3g; Protein: 3g; Carbohydrates: 9g; Fiber: 3g; Sugar: 2g

Per serving (Cinnamon Sugar, ¼ cup): Calories: 84; Fat: 3g; Protein: 3g; Carbohydrates: 12g; Fiber: 3g; Sugar: 5g

Per serving (Barbecue, ¼ cup): Calories: 71; Fat: 3g; Protein: 3g; Carbohydrates: 9g; Fiber: 3g; Sugar: 2g

Per serving (Salty and Spicy, ¼ cup): Calories: 70; Fat: 3g; Protein: 3g; Carbohydrates: 9g; Fiber: 2g; Sugar: 2g

Flaxseed Chips and Guacamole

Prep time: 10 minutes / Cook time: 1 hour / Serves 6

GLUTEN-FREE

For the crackers

1 cup flaxseed

½ cup Vegetable
  Broth (page 134)
  or store-bought

2 teaspoons garlic powder

2 teaspoons paprika

1 teaspoon onion salt

2 teaspoons onion powder

For the guacamole

3 large avocados, halved
  and pitted

½ cup diced red onion

1 tablespoon lime juice

½ teaspoon salt

¼ teaspoon
  ground cumin

To make the crackers

1. Preheat the oven to 325°F. Line a baking sheet with parchment paper.

2. In a large mixing bowl, mix together the flaxseed, broth, garlic powder, paprika, onion salt, and onion powder until well combined.

3. Spread the mixture in a thin, even layer on the prepared baking sheet and bake for 55 to 60 minutes, until slightly crispy on the edges. Let the baked flaxseed sheet cool before breaking it into chip-size pieces.

To make the guacamole

4. In a medium mixing bowl, mash the avocados well with the back of a fork.

5. Add the red onion, lime juice, salt, and cumin and mix to combine. Cover and refrigerate until ready to eat.

Love your leftovers: The crackers can be stored in an airtight container or a zip-top bag at room temperature for up to one week.

Per serving (½ cup guac and 12 chips): Calories: 353; Fat: 28g; Protein: 9g; Carbohydrates: 24g; Fiber: 17g; Sugar: 5g

Coconut Brownie Truffles

Prep time: 15 minutes / Makes 20 truffles

½ cup unsweetened coconut

¼ cup brown rice syrup

2 tablespoons coconut oil, melted

½ cup natural almond butter

1 teaspoon coconut extract

1 cup oat flour

3 tablespoons unsweetened cocoa powder

2½ tablespoons (1 scoop) vanilla or chocolate vegan protein powder

¼ cup dairy-free dark chocolate chips, roughly chopped

1. Line a baking sheet with parchment paper or aluminum foil.

2. In a food processor or high-powered blender, pulse the coconut until it is broken down into fine pieces. Set aside.

3. In the bowl of a stand mixer, beat the brown rice syrup, coconut oil, almond butter, coconut extract, oat flour, cocoa powder, and protein powder on medium speed until well combined. If mixing by hand, stir well with a spatula until all the ingredients are combined to form a batter.

4. Add the chocolate chips and beat until they are just incorporated.

5. Add the shredded coconut and beat until it is just incorporated.

6. Roll the mixture into 1-inch balls and set them on the prepared baking sheet.

7. Place the baking sheet in the refrigerator and chill for about 1 hour, until set. Serve immediately or store them in an airtight container in the refrigerator until ready to eat.

 Love your leftovers: The truffles can be frozen for up to two weeks. To defrost them, leave the truffles at room temperature for 10 to 15 minutes, until soft.

 Smart shopping: I recommend IdealRaw Protein Powder, which is vegan and doesn't contain any artificial sweeteners. For the dairy-free chocolate chips, I recommend Lily's, which are sweetened with stevia and gluten-free.

Per serving (2 truffles): Calories: 243; Fat: 16g; Protein: 7g; Carbohydrates: 23g; Fiber: 5g; Sugar: 6g

Double Chocolate Peanut Butter Cookies

Prep time: 15 minutes, plus 30 minutes to chill / Makes 40 cookies

NO COOK

GLUTEN-FREE OPTION

3 cups quick (or gluten-free) oats

1 cup coarsely chopped almonds

3 tablespoons unsweetened cocoa powder

½ cup coconut oil

1 cup natural peanut butter, chunky

¼ cup brown rice syrup

2 teaspoons vanilla extract

⅛ teaspoon salt

½ cup dairy-free dark chocolate chips

1. Line a baking sheet with parchment paper or aluminum foil.

2. In a medium bowl, whisk together the quick oats, almonds, and cocoa powder. Set aside.

3. In a small saucepan over medium-low heat, combine the coconut oil and peanut butter. Cook for 3 to 4 minutes, until melted and smooth. Remove the saucepan from the heat. Add the brown rice syrup, vanilla, salt, and dark chocolate chips and cook, stirring, until melted and combined.

4. Add the chocolate mixture into the oat mixture and stir to combine.

5. Using a small cookie scoop, form 40 small balls and place them on the prepared baking sheet. Refrigerate for about 30 minutes, until hardened.

 Love your leftovers: Store the cookies in an airtight container in the refrigerator for up to seven days.

 Smart shopping: For the dairy-free chocolate chips, I recommend Lily's, which are sweetened with stevia and gluten-free. For the peanut butter, I recommend Adams, which is all-natural and only contains peanuts and a tiny bit of salt.

Per serving (2 cookies): Calories: 250; Fat: 18g; Protein: 7g; Carbohydrates: 20g; Fiber: 5g; Sugar: 4g

Brownie Batter Hummus

Prep time: 10 minutes / Serves 6

1 (15-ounce) can chickpeas, drained and rinsed

2 tablespoons almond butter

1/3 cup unsweetened cocoa powder

1/4 cup maple syrup

1/2 teaspoon salt

1 teaspoon vanilla extract

1/3 cup unsweetened almond milk

1/4 cup dairy-free dark chocolate chips, roughly chopped

Apple slices, for pairing (optional)

Strawberries, for pairing (optional)

Pretzels, for pairing (optional)

1. In a food processor or high-powered blender, combine the chickpeas and almond butter and pulse for about 1 minute, until the beans are a paste-like texture.

2. Add the cocoa powder, maple syrup, salt, and vanilla and pulse again for about 1 minute. Add the almond milk, a little bit at a time, and blend until incorporated.

3. Add the chocolate chips and blend for about 1 minute, until everything is incorporated.

4. Using a spatula, transfer the mixture to a small serving bowl, scraping down the sides of the blender, and serve with apple slices, strawberries, or pretzels (if using).

ONE POT

NO COOK

GLUTEN-FREE

 Smart shopping: For the dairy-free chocolate chips, I recommend Lily's, which are sweetened with stevia and gluten-free.

Per serving (¼ cup): Calories: 163; Fat: 7g; Protein: 6g; Carbohydrates: 26g; Fiber: 7g; Sugar: 11g

Chunky Monkey Nice Cream

Prep time: 10 minutes / Serves 1

QUICK

ONE POT

NO COOK

GLUTEN-FREE

5-INGREDIENT

1 medium banana, frozen and cut into thirds

2½ tablespoons (1 scoop) vegan chocolate peanut butter protein powder

2 to 3 tablespoons dairy-free milk of choice

1 tablespoon natural peanut butter

1. In a high-powered blender, pulse the frozen banana until creamy.

2. Add the protein powder and pulse until fully incorporated. Slowly add the dairy-free milk and pulse until the mixture is a bit thinner.

3. Stir in the peanut butter by hand until combined.

4. Transfer the mixture into a bowl and eat immediately, or if you like a firmer texture, freeze for 5 minutes, or until it is slightly harder than soft-serve ice cream.

 Smart shopping: I recommend IdealRaw Protein Powder, which is vegan and doesn't contain any artificial sweeteners. For the peanut butter, I recommend Adams, which is all-natural and only contains peanuts and a tiny bit of salt.

Per serving: Calories: 336; Fat: 14g; Protein: 20g; Carbohydrates: 40g; Fiber: 8g; Sugar: 18g

Granola Pumpkin Seed Bars

Prep time: 15 minutes / Cook time: 30 minutes / Makes 12 bars

Nonstick cooking spray

½ cup pumpkin seeds

½ cup chia seeds

¾ cup golden raisins

⅔ cup almond flour

¼ cup granulated monk
fruit sweetener

2 tablespoons coconut
oil, melted

1 tablespoon
vanilla extract

½ cup brown rice syrup

¼ teaspoon salt

1. Preheat the oven to 320°F. Spray a 9-by-13-inch baking pan with nonstick cooking spray and set it aside.

2. In a medium bowl, mix together the pumpkin seeds, chia seeds, raisins, and almond flour. Set aside.

3. In medium saucepan over medium-low heat, combine the monk fruit sweetener, coconut oil, vanilla, brown rice syrup, and salt. Bring to a simmer and cook, stirring occasionally, for 2 to 3 minutes. Pour the mixture over the pumpkin seed mixture and stir until well incorporated.

4. Spread the mixture evenly into the prepared baking pan. Press the mixture down firmly with the back of a spatula.

5. Bake for 25 minutes, until lightly browned

6. Let it cool before cutting into 12 portions. The bars will harden as they cool.

 Love your leftovers: These bars can be individually wrapped and stored at room temperature for up to seven days.

 Smart shopping: Granulated monk fruit sweetener is an all-natural sweetener derived from dried fruit. It's extremely potent, so you don't need to use as much. It has no calories and no effect on blood sugar. It can easily be found in the baking aisle of most grocery stores.

Per serving (1 bar): Calories: 204; Fat: 10g; Protein: 4g; Carbohydrates: 25g; Fiber: 5g; Sugar: 14g

Churro Popcorn

Prep time: 5 minutes / Cook time: 5 minutes / Serves 5

SOY-FREE

QUICK

GLUTEN-FREE

5-INGREDIENT

1 cup popcorn kernels

3 tablespoons coconut oil, plus 2 teaspoons

½ teaspoon salt, divided

1 teaspoon coconut sugar

1 teaspoon ground cinnamon

1. In a large stockpot over medium-high heat, combine the popcorn kernels and 3 tablespoons of coconut oil. Sprinkle it with ¼ teaspoon of salt, cover, and gently shake the pan back and forth over the heat for about 3 minutes, until the popcorn pops. Once the popping slows, remove the pot from the heat and set aside.

2. In a small saucepan over medium-high heat, mix together the remaining 2 teaspoons of coconut oil, the coconut sugar, cinnamon, and the remaining ¼ teaspoon of salt and simmer for 1 minute.

3. Pour the topping over the popcorn and quickly stir to combine.

Love your leftovers: The popcorn can be stored in an airtight container for up to five days.

Variation tip: Feel free to experiment with flavors and ingredients. You could make it a savory popcorn by adding some garlic salt and cumin instead of the coconut sugar and cinnamon. Make sure to heat up the spices before pouring them over the popcorn for a richer flavor and aroma!

Per serving (2 cups): Calories: 264; Fat: 12g; Protein: 5g; Carbohydrates: 35g; Fiber: 6g; Sugar: 1g

Apple Nachos

Prep time: 10 minutes / Cook time: 2 to 3 minutes / Serves 1

1 apple, cored and thinly sliced

¼ cup dairy-free dark chocolate chips

½ tablespoon almond butter

½ tablespoon coconut oil

Chopped almonds, for topping (optional)

Unsweetened coconut flakes, for topping (optional)

Sunflower seeds, for topping (optional)

1. Arrange the apple slices on a plate.

2. Place the chocolate chips in a medium microwave-safe bowl and microwave in 30-second intervals, stirring between each interval, until completely melted.

3. In another small microwave-safe bowl, combine the almond butter and coconut oil and microwave until soft, but not completely melted.

4. Drizzle the apple slices with the chocolate mixture, and then with the almond butter mixture. Sprinkle them with your favorite toppings (if using) and serve.

Smart shopping: For the dairy-free chocolate chips, I recommend Lily's, which are sweetened with stevia and gluten-free.

Variation tip: I prefer using a Honeycrisp or Fuji apple, but Granny Smiths are good if you want a tart contrast to the sweetness of the topping.

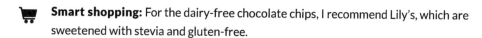

Per serving (1 apple): Calories: 323; Fat: 21g; Protein: 4g; Carbohydrates: 45g; Fiber: 13g; Sugar: 21g

Lemon-Chia Powerbites

Prep time: 12 minutes, plus 30 minutes to chill / Makes 14 powerbites

½ cup unsweetened coconut flakes

½ cup quick oats

2 tablespoons chia seeds, divided

3 cups vegan vanilla protein powder

1 tablespoon coconut sugar

1 teaspoon lemon zest

4 tablespoons lemon juice

1. Line a baking sheet with parchment paper or aluminum foil.

2. In a high-powered blender or food processor, combine the coconut, quick oats, and 1 tablespoon of the chia seeds and pulse a few times, until the mixture becomes powderlike. Transfer it to a plate and set aside.

3. In a small bowl, mix together the protein powder, coconut sugar, lemon zest, and the remaining 1 tablespoon of chia seeds.

4. Add the lemon juice and 6 tablespoons of water and stir until combined.

5. Form the mixture into 14 balls. Roll the balls in the coconut mixture to coat, place them on the prepared baking sheet, and put them in the freezer for 30 minutes.

6. Remove the balls from the freezer and store them in an airtight container in the refrigerator for up to 5 days.

Love your leftovers: Store these powerbites in the freezer for up to three months. To thaw, place on the counter for about five minutes before enjoying.

Smart shopping: I recommend IdealRaw Protein Powder, which is vegan and doesn't contain any artificial sweeteners.

Technique tip: Depending on the protein powder you use, you may need to add more water, since they vary in terms of dryness.

Per serving (2 powerbites): Calories: 414; Fat: 19g; Protein: 43g; Carbohydrates: 20g; Fiber: 6g; Sugar: 8g

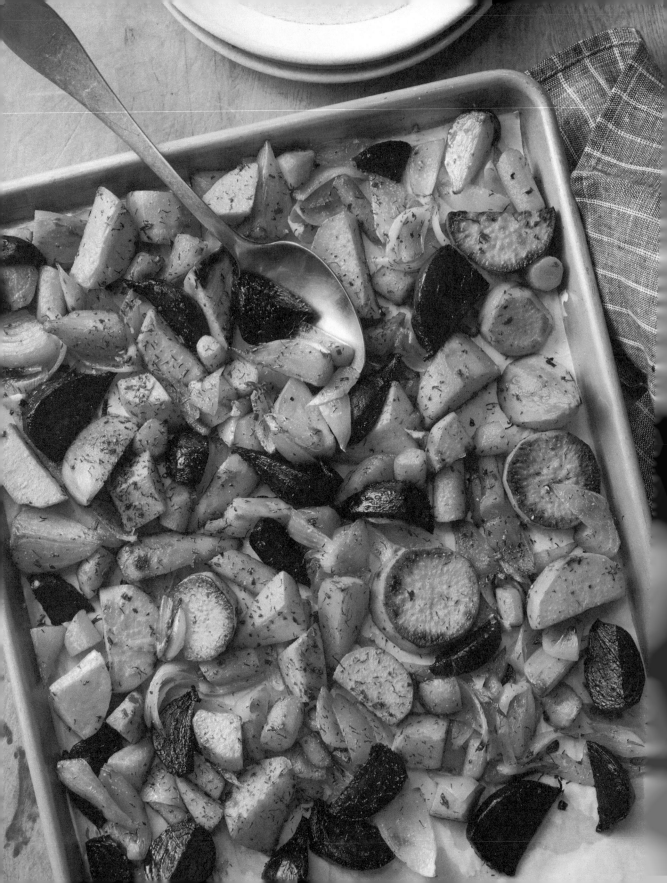

CHAPTER 7

Batch Cook Basics

< Roasted Root Vegetables, page 125

Refried Beans

Prep time: 8 to 10 hours / Cook time: 2 to 3 hours / Serves 7

SOY-FREE

ONE POT

NUT-FREE

GLUTEN-FREE

5-INGREDIENT

3 cups dried pinto beans

1 to 2 teaspoons salt

1. Rinse the beans thoroughly and remove any stones.

2. Place the beans in a large bowl, cover them completely with water, and cover the bowl with a dish towel. Soak at room temperature for 8 to 10 hours or overnight.

3. Drain the beans and pour them into a large stockpot over medium-high heat. Add 6 cups of water and bring to a boil. Reduce the heat to medium-low, cover, and simmer, checking the beans for doneness every 45 minutes, for 2 to 3 hours, until very tender.

4. Strain the beans in a colander set over a large bowl and reserve the liquid.

5. Transfer the beans back into the stockpot and mash them with a potato masher. Add in the reserved bean liquid, ½ cup at a time, as you mash until they are the consistency of refried beans. Add 1 teaspoon of salt and stir to combine. Taste and add the remaining 1 teaspoon of salt if desired.

 Appliance tip: If you have an Instant Pot, cooking these beans is a breeze. Place the beans and 6 cups of water in the Instant Pot and cook on high pressure for 50 minutes. Release the pressure naturally for 10 minutes. Continue following the recipe above at step 4 to finish the recipe.

 Love your leftovers: These beans are so flavorful and versatile, especially for the vegan diet. You can use them in burritos, tacos, or even paired with some tofu and fajita vegetables. You can also use them instead of black beans in my Tex-Mex Enchilada Bake (page 92) and Easy Mediterranean Quesadilla (page 74).

Per serving (½ cup): Calories: 287; Fat: 1g; Protein: 18g; Carbohydrates: 52g; Fiber: 13g; Sugar: 2g

Easy Lentils

Prep time: 10 minutes / Cook time: 25 minutes / Serves 8

1½ cups brown or
green lentils

1 tablespoon olive oil

½ medium onion,
finely diced

2 garlic cloves, minced

5 cups Vegetable
Broth (page 134)
or store-bought

1 teaspoon dried oregano

1 bay leaf

¼ teaspoon
salt (optional)

1. Rinse the lentils in a colander and remove any stones. Set aside.

2. In a large saucepan over medium-high heat, warm the olive oil. Add the onion and sauté, stirring, for about 3 minutes. Add the garlic and cook for about 1 minute, until fragrant.

3. Add the broth, oregano, bay leaf, and lentils and bring to a boil, stirring frequently. Reduce the heat to medium-low and simmer for about 20 minutes, until tender but not falling apart.

4. Remove and discard the bay leaf and drain the lentils in a colander.

5. Return the lentils to the saucepan and season them with the salt (if using).

 Cooking tip: Lentils are a wonderful source of plant-based protein, and they're also high in fiber. Feel free to add them to salads, soups, or bowls.

 Love your leftovers: To store the lentils, place them in an airtight container in the refrigerator for up to seven days, or seal them in a gallon-size zip-top bag in the freezer for up to three months.

Per serving (½ cup): Calories: 182; Fat: 5g; Protein: 9g; Carbohydrates: 26g; Fiber: 5g; Sugar: 2g

SOY-FREE / ONE POT / NUT-FREE / GLUTEN-FREE

Perfect Quinoa

Prep time: 5 minutes / Cook time: 20 minutes / Serves 4

SOY-FREE

QUICK

ONE POT

NUT-FREE

GLUTEN-FREE

5-INGREDIENT

1 cup quinoa

1 teaspoon olive oil

1 garlic clove, minced

2 tablespoons minced flat leaf parsley

1¾ cups Vegetable Broth (page 134) or store-bought

1. Place the quinoa in a fine mesh sieve and rinse very well, which will remove any bitter taste. Set aside.

2. In a small saucepan over medium heat, warm the olive oil. Add the garlic and sauté for 1 to 2 minutes, until fragrant.

3. Add the parsley, vegetable broth, and quinoa, stir to combine, and bring to a boil. Reduce the heat to low, cover, and cook for 15 minutes. Remove the saucepan from the heat and let it rest for 10 minutes.

4. Remove the lid and fluff the quinoa with a fork.

Ingredient tip: There are several different types of quinoa. White quinoa is better for stir-fries and bowls, while red quinoa is denser and holds up better in salads.

Per serving (½ cup): Calories: 193; Fat: 6g; Protein: 6g; Carbohydrates: 29g; Fiber: 4g; Sugar: 3g

Tabbouleh

Prep time: 15 minutes, plus 1 hour to chill / Serves 9

1 cup Perfect Quinoa
(page 122)

3 cups chopped parsley

2 cups seeded and
chopped Roma tomatoes

2 cups peeled and
diced cucumber

½ cup finely diced
red onion

½ cup chopped fresh
mint leaves

Juice of 1 lime

1 teaspoon salt

½ cup olive oil

Freshly ground
black pepper

1. In a large serving bowl, mix together the quinoa, parsley, tomatoes, cucumber, onion, and mint.

2. In a small bowl, mix together the lime juice, salt, and olive oil.

3. Pour the dressing over the salad and stir well.

4. Top the salad with pepper to taste and cover it with plastic wrap.

5. Refrigerate for at least 1 hour before serving.

 Cooking tip: Tabbouleh is typically made with bulgur, but quinoa is a great swap. Not only is it easier to find in stores, but it also makes the dish gluten-free.

 Love your leftovers: To store the tabbouleh, place it in an airtight container in the refrigerator for up to four days. Tabbouleh pairs nicely with my Baked Falafel Salad (page 64) and Toasted Lavash and Chickpea Salad (page 66).

Per serving (1 cup): Calories: 160; Fat: 13g; Protein: 3g; Carbohydrates: 10g; Fiber: 2g; Sugar: 2g

SOY-FREE

ONE POT

NUT-FREE

NO COOK

GLUTEN-FREE

Cauliflower Tots

Prep time: 15 minutes / Cook time: 30 minutes / Serves 6

SOY-FREE

1 tablespoon flaxseed

2½ cups riced cauliflower

1 tablespoon olive oil

¼ cup diced onion

3 garlic cloves,
   finely minced

½ cup panko
   bread crumbs

1 teaspoon dried parsley

1 teaspoon salt

¼ cup shredded
   dairy-free cheese

1. Preheat the oven to 450°F. Line a baking sheet with aluminum foil and set it aside.

2. In a small bowl, mix the flaxseed with 3 tablespoons of water. Place the mixture in the refrigerator for 15 minutes, until thickened.

3. Cook the riced cauliflower according to the package instructions. Drain well.

4. While the cauliflower is cooking: In a small skillet over medium heat, warm the olive oil. Add the onion and garlic and sauté for about 3 minutes. Set aside to cool.

5. In a large bowl, mix together the bread crumbs, parsley, and salt. Add the cauliflower rice and the sautéed onion and garlic. Stir well. Add the cheese and stir to combine.

6. Form the cauliflower mixture, 1½ to 2 tablespoons at a time, into tots. Place the tots on the prepared baking sheet and bake for 15 minutes. Flip each tot and continue baking for 10 to 12 minutes, until the tops are golden brown.

7. Let the tots cool slightly before serving.

 Smart shopping: I like the flavor of Daiya brand dairy-free cheese.

 Love your leftovers: Serve any leftovers alongside my Lemon Pepper Tofu Steak with Broccoli (page 95) or Kale Caesar Salad (page 62). Sometimes, I even add Cauliflower Tots to my Green Goddess Buddha Bowl (page 90).

Per serving (8 tots): Calories: 76; Fat: 4g; Protein: 2g; Carbohydrates: 10g; Fiber: 2g; Sugar: 1g

Roasted Root Vegetables

Prep time: 10 minutes / Cook time: 25 minutes / Serves 4

1 cup roughly
chopped onion

1 cup peeled and
chopped carrots

1 cup peeled and chopped
sweet potatoes

1 cup peeled and
chopped beets

2 tablespoons olive oil

¼ cup Clean Ranch
Seasoning (page 137)

1. Preheat the oven to 425°F. Line a baking sheet with aluminum foil and set it aside.

2. In a medium bowl, mix together the onion, carrots, sweet potatoes, and beets. Pour the olive oil over the vegetables and toss well.

3. Add the ranch seasoning and stir with a spatula until the vegetables are well coated.

4. Spread the vegetables in a single layer onto the prepared baking sheet and bake for 12 minutes. Stir the vegetables and bake for another 12 minutes, until they are brown and bubbly.

 Love your leftovers: If plant-based eating is new for you, then you will love making these roasted root veggies. You can enjoy these for really any meal of the day. Try pairing them with my Green Goddess Buddha Bowl (page 90) or using them in my Chipotle Breakfast Burrito (page 56) or as one of the fixings for my Cauliflower Tacos (page 94).

Per serving (½ cup vegetables): Calories: 192; Fat: 7g; Protein: 4g; Carbohydrates: 30g; Fiber: 6g; Sugar: 12g

SOY-FREE

NUT-FREE

GLUTEN-FREE

5-INGREDIENT

Sweet Potato Steaks

Prep time: 5 minutes / Cook time: 20 minutes / Serves 8

SOY-FREE

QUICK

ONE POT

NUT-FREE

GLUTEN-FREE

5-INGREDIENT

2 large sweet
   potatoes, scrubbed

Nonstick cooking spray

1 teaspoon sea salt

1. Preheat the oven to 400°F. Place a wire rack on
   a baking sheet (if you don't have a wire rack,
   you can line the baking sheet with parchment
   paper instead).

2. Trim the ends off the sweet potatoes. Using a
   sharp knife or mandolin, cut the sweet potatoes
   lengthwise into ¼-inch-thick slices.

3. Arrange the sliced potatoes in a single layer on the
   wire rack. Spray the sweet potatoes lightly with
   nonstick cooking spray and sprinkle them with the
   sea salt.

4. Bake for 20 minutes. Let the sweet potato steaks
   cool for 10 minutes.

5. To reheat the sweet potato steaks, place them in a
   toaster oven and toast until heated through.

 Cooking tip: Leaving the peel on the sweet potatoes makes the steaks sturdier, and they
will hold up better if you add toppings.

 Love your leftovers: These sweet potato steaks can be stored in an airtight container in
the refrigerator for up to seven days. Having these on hand will be a big time saver; they
can be diced up to use in other recipes that call for sweet potatoes, such as my Chipotle
Breakfast Burrito (page 56).

Per serving (2 slices): Calories: 45; Fat: 0g; Protein: 1g; Carbohydrates: 10g; Fiber: 2g;
Sugar: 2g

Coconut-Cilantro Rice

Prep time: 10 minutes / Cook time: 25 minutes / Serves 8

2 cups basmati rice

1 (13.5-ounce) can light
coconut milk

3 tablespoons
chopped cilantro

1 teaspoon salt

2 teaspoons
coconut sugar

1. In a medium saucepan over high heat, mix together
the rice, coconut milk, cilantro, salt, coconut
sugar, and 2 cups of water and bring it to a boil,
stirring frequently.

2. Reduce the heat to low, cover, and cook for
25 minutes, until tender.

3. Remove the saucepan from the heat and fluff the
rice with a fork.

 Cooking tip: If you are using regular white rice, reduce the cooking time by five minutes.

 Love your leftovers: This flavorful dish is a great option to add to any plant-based meal.
Feel free to serve it alongside my Lemon Pepper Tofu Steak with Broccoli (page 95), in my
Green Goddess Buddha Bowl (page 90), or in place of quinoa in my Black Bean and Sweet
Potato Tortilla Soup (page 100).

Per serving (½ cup): Calories: 211; Fat: 3g; Protein: 4g; Carbohydrates: 40g; Fiber: 0g;
Sugar: 1g

SOY-FREE

ONE POT

GLUTEN-FREE

5-INGREDIENT

Roasted Brussels Sprouts

Prep time: 10 minutes / Cook time: 25 minutes / Serves 5

SOY-FREE

ONE POT

NUT-FREE

GLUTEN-FREE

5-INGREDIENT

1 pound Brussels sprouts, trimmed and halved

1½ tablespoons olive oil

1 teaspoon garlic powder

1 teaspoon salt

¼ teaspoon freshly ground black pepper

1. Preheat the oven to 425°F. Line a baking sheet with aluminum foil and set it aside.

2. In a medium bowl, toss the Brussels sprouts with the olive oil until coated well.

3. Add the garlic powder, salt, and pepper and toss again. Spread the sprouts in a single layer on the prepared baking sheet.

4. Roast for 12 minutes. Toss the Brussels sprouts with a spatula and continue roasting for 12 to 14 more minutes, until the tops are golden brown and slightly crispy.

Technique tip: If your Brussels sprouts ever taste bitter after roasting, it means they are overcooked. Make sure to keep an eye on them in the last few minutes of roasting to ensure that they don't get too brown.

Per serving (1 cup): Calories: 77; Fat: 4g; Protein: 3g; Carbohydrates: 9g; Fiber: 4g; Sugar: 2g

Quick and Easy Pickled Cabbage

Prep time: 10 minutes, plus 4 hours to sit / Makes 4 (16-ounce) jars

1 small head red cabbage, cored and cut into thin strips

½ cup red wine vinegar

½ cup apple cider vinegar

4 tablespoons coconut sugar

2 garlic cloves, minced

1 teaspoon salt

⅛ teaspoon freshly ground black pepper

SOY-FREE
NO COOK
GLUTEN-FREE
5-INGREDIENT

1. Divide the cabbage between 4 (16-ounce) glass jars (with lids), making sure to leave ½ inch at the top of each jar.

2. In a medium bowl, mix together the red wine vinegar, apple cider vinegar, coconut sugar, and 1 cup of water until the sugar is dissolved.

3. Add the garlic, salt, and pepper and stir to combine.

4. Pour the liquid equally into each jar, covering the cabbage. If you don't have enough liquid to cover all the jars, fill them up three-quarters of the way. As the cabbage softens, it will compress into the liquid.

5. Cover the jars and let them sit at room temperature for at least 4 hours before serving.

Variation tip: Use this same method to pickle other vegetables, such as carrots and onions. Add the pickled vegetables to any vegan dish, such as avocado toast, a Buddha bowl, or a simple stir-fry.

Love your leftovers: This pickled cabbage can be refrigerated for up to two weeks. Not only are fermented veggies good for your gut, they also add great flavor and texture to any salad. I love them in my Green Goddess Buddha Bowl (page 90), but they can be added to any meal. This cabbage would also be delicious with my Baked Falafel Salad (page 64) or inside my Loaded Bell Pepper Sandwich (page 69).

Per serving (2 tablespoons): Calories: 103; Fat: <1g; Protein: 2g; Carbohydrates: 23g; Fiber: 3g; Sugar: 18g

Roasted Spaghetti Squash

Prep time: 10 minutes / Cook time: 50 minutes / Serves 4

SOY-FREE

NUT-FREE

GLUTEN-FREE

5-INGREDIENT

1 spaghetti squash

2 tablespoons olive oil

1 teaspoon salt

¼ teaspoon freshly
ground black pepper

1. Preheat the oven to 400°F. Line a baking sheet with aluminum foil.

2. Trim the ends off of the spaghetti squash and cut it in half lengthwise. Scoop out and discard the seeds.

3. Rub 1 tablespoon of the olive oil over the cut side of each squash half. Sprinkle the squash halves with the salt and pepper and place them facedown on the prepared baking sheet.

4. Roast for 35 to 50 minutes, or until the flesh is tender.

5. When the squash is cool enough to handle, use a fork to gently scrape out the flesh, releasing spaghetti-like strands.

 Love your leftovers: Store this "spaghetti" in an airtight container in the refrigerator for up to four days.

Per serving (1 cup): Calories: 112; Fat: 7g; Protein: 1g; Carbohydrates: 13g; Fiber: 3g; Sugar: 5g

Marinated Tofu

Prep time: 5 minutes, plus 1 hour to chill / Cook time: 30 minutes / Serves 4

1 (14-ounce) package extra-firm lite tofu, pressed and drained

Juice of 2 lemons

3 tablespoons avocado oil

1 tablespoon Dijon mustard

3 garlic cloves, smashed

1 tablespoon dried oregano

¼ teaspoon salt

1. Cut the tofu into 1-inch cubes and set aside.

2. In a gallon-size zip-top bag, mix together the lemon juice, avocado oil, Dijon mustard, garlic, oregano, and salt. Add the tofu, seal the bag, and gently toss to coat the tofu pieces.

3. Refrigerate for at least 1 hour but preferably overnight. This will result in the best flavor possible for the tofu.

4. Preheat the oven to 400°F. Line a baking sheet with aluminum foil or parchment paper.

5. Drain and discard the marinade and place the tofu on the prepared baking sheet.

6. Bake for 15 minutes, flip the tofu, and bake for an additional 15 minutes, or until the tofu is slightly browned.

 Love your leftovers: To store the tofu, place it in an airtight container or zip-top bag in the refrigerator for up to four days. It's always a good idea to have this recipe prepped and ready for easy meal assembly. This can be used alongside roasted vegetables or in my Green Goddess Buddha Bowl (page 90) or Cashew and Tofu Stir-Fry (page 88).

Per serving (4 oz): Calories: 180; Fat: 13g; Protein: 9g; Carbohydrates: 7g; Fiber: 2g; Sugar: 1g

ONE POT

NUT-FREE

GLUTEN-FREE

5-INGREDIENT

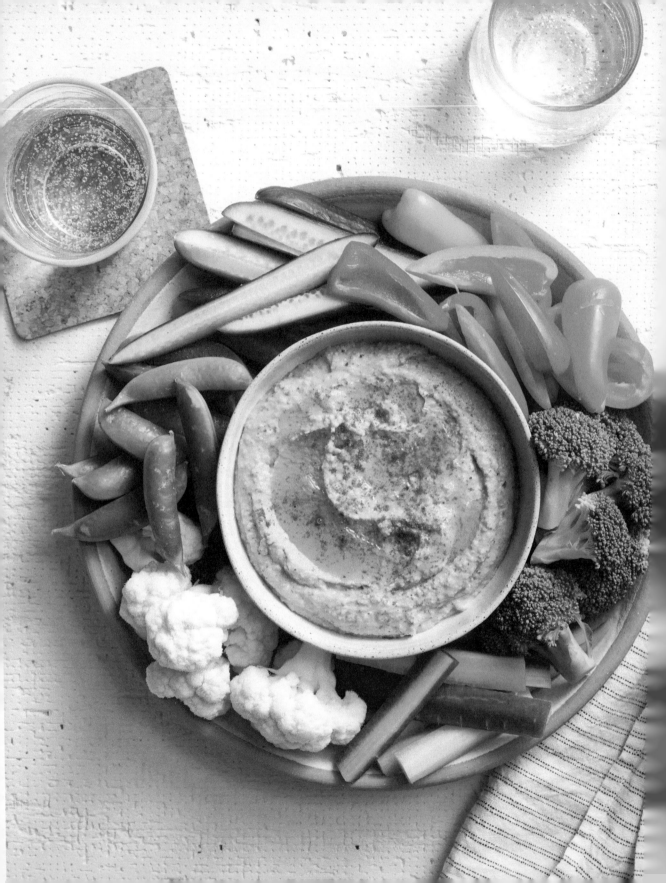

Homemade Staples

< Not-So-Spicy Jalapeño Hummus, page 144

Vegetable Broth

Prep time: 15 minutes / Cook time: 1 hour 10 minutes / Makes 6 cups

SOY-FREE

ONE POT

NUT-FREE

GLUTEN-FREE

2 tablespoons olive oil

2 onions,
    roughly chopped

3 garlic cloves, smashed

1 tablespoon tomato paste

4 celery stalks, cut into
    1-inch pieces

2 carrots,
    roughly chopped

1 teaspoon salt

½ teaspoon freshly
    ground black pepper

3 tablespoons chopped
    fresh parsley

1 thyme sprig

1 bay leaf

1. In a large stockpot over medium-high heat, warm the olive oil. Add the onions and sauté for about 4 minutes. Add the garlic and stir for 1 minute.

2. Add the tomato paste and stir until combined. Add 6 cups of water and cook, stirring, for 1 or 2 more minutes.

3. Add the celery, carrots, salt, pepper, parsley, thyme, and bay leaf and bring to a boil. Reduce the heat to low, cover, and simmer for 1 hour.

4. Using a fine mesh sieve over a large bowl, strain the broth and let it cool.

5. Use the broth immediately or store it in airtight containers or zip-top bags in the refrigerator for up to 7 days.

 Love your leftovers: This broth freezes wonderfully for up to four months. Store it in zip-top bags and lay them flat in the freezer. To defrost, transfer the bags to the refrigerator or run them under warm water until they thaw.

Per serving (1 cup): Calories: 57; Fat: 5g; Protein: 1g; Carbohydrates: 4g; Fiber: 1g; Sugar: 2g

Vegan Parmesan

Prep time: 5 minutes / Makes 6 tablespoons

½ cup raw almonds

2 tablespoons
  nutritional yeast

½ teaspoon salt

¼ teaspoon garlic powder

In a blender, combine the almonds, yeast, salt, and garlic powder and blend until it is a smooth, grated cheese–like texture. Do not over-blend.

 Love your leftovers: Store this vegan Parmesan in an airtight container in the refrigerator for up to one month. Add it to any vegan dish that calls for non-dairy Parmesan cheese.

Per serving (2 tablespoons): Calories: 146; Fat: 11g; Protein: 8g; Carbohydrates: 7g; Fiber: 4g; Sugar: 1g

SOY-FREE

QUICK

NO COOK

GLUTEN-FREE

5-INGREDIENT

Vegan Mayo

Prep time: 7 minutes / Makes 1 cup

QUICK

ONE POT

NUT-FREE

NO COOK

GLUTEN-FREE

5-INGREDIENT

1 (14-ounce) package extra-firm lite tofu

Juice of 1 lemon

1 tablespoon white vinegar

1½ teaspoons Dijon mustard

¼ teaspoon salt

¼ teaspoon onion powder

1. In a food processor or high-powered blender, combine the tofu, lemon juice, vinegar, mustard, salt, and onion powder and blend on high for 3 to 4 minutes, until smooth.

2. Scrape down the sides of the processor or blender and blend again for about 1 minute.

Love your leftovers: Store the mayo in an airtight container in the refrigerator for up to five days.

Variation tip: If you want to spice this mayo up a bit, add garlic powder and two chipotle peppers to make it a chipotle aioli.

Per serving (2 tablespoons): Calories: 41; Fat: 1g; Protein: 5g; Carbohydrates: 2g; Fiber: 1g; Sugar: <1g

Clean Ranch Seasoning

Prep time: 5 minutes / Makes 2 tablespoons

½ teaspoon dried chives

½ teaspoon dried parsley

½ teaspoon dried
dill weed

¼ teaspoon garlic powder

¼ teaspoon
onion powder

⅛ teaspoon salt

⅛ teaspoon freshly
ground black pepper

1. In a zip-top bag, mix together the chives, parsley, dill, garlic powder, onion powder, salt, and pepper.

2. Seal the bag and store it at room temperature until ready to use.

 Cooking tip: Two tablespoons of seasoning mix is equal to one packet of store-bought ranch seasoning.

Per serving (2 tablespoons): Calories: 7; Fat: <1g; Protein: <1g; Carbohydrates: 2g; Fiber: <1g; Sugar: <1g

SOY-FREE

QUICK

NUT-FREE

NO COOK

GLUTEN-FREE

5-INGREDIENT

Taco Seasoning

Prep time: 2 minutes / Makes about ½ cup

SOY-FREE

QUICK

NUT-FREE

NO COOK

GLUTEN-FREE

6 tablespoons
chili powder

1 tablespoon oregano

4 teaspoons
ground cumin

3 teaspoons paprika

2 teaspoons garlic powder

1 teaspoon freshly ground
black pepper

1 teaspoon salt

½ teaspoon
cayenne pepper

In a small bowl, mix together the chili powder, oregano, cumin, paprika, garlic powder, black pepper, salt, and cayenne. Transfer the seasoning to an airtight container, and store it at room temperature for up to 3 months.

Per serving (2 tablespoons): Calories: 55; Fat: 2g; Protein: 3g; Carbohydrates: 10g; Fiber: 6g; Sugar: 0g

Garam Masala

Prep time: 2 minutes / Makes about ¼ cup

2 tablespoons
  ground coriander

1 tablespoon
  ground cumin

½ teaspoon freshly
  ground black pepper

¾ teaspoon
  ground cinnamon

½ teaspoon
  ground cloves

½ teaspoon
  ground cardamom

¼ teaspoon nutmeg

In a small bowl, mix together the coriander, cumin, pepper, cinnamon, cloves, cardamom, and nutmeg. Transfer the spice blend to an airtight container, and store it at room temperature for up to 2 months.

Per serving (2 tablespoons): Calories: 25; Fat: 1g; Protein: 1g; Carbohydrates: 4g; Fiber: 2g; Sugar: <1g

SOY-FREE

QUICK

NUT-FREE

NO COOK

GLUTEN-FREE

Everything Bagel Seasoning

Prep time: 2 minutes / Makes about ¼ cup

SOY-FREE

QUICK

NUT-FREE

NO COOK

GLUTEN-FREE

5-INGREDIENT

2 tablespoons white
sesame seeds

1 tablespoon black
sesame seeds

1 tablespoon dried
minced onion

1 tablespoon garlic salt

1½ teaspoons
poppy seeds

In a small bowl, mix together the white and black sesame seeds, dried onion, garlic salt, and poppy seeds. Transfer the seasoning blend to an airtight container, and store it at room temperature for up to 2 months.

Per serving (1 tablespoon): Calories: 57; Fat: 5g; Protein: 2g; Carbohydrates: 3g; Fiber: 1g; Sugar: 1g

Lemon Tahini Dressing

Prep time: 10 minutes / Makes 2 cups

Juice of 1 lemon

2 tablespoons olive oil

2 garlic cloves

½ cup tahini

½ red bell pepper, seeded

¼ white onion

½ teaspoon salt

½ teaspoon freshly
   ground black pepper

In a high-powered blender, combine the lemon juice, olive oil, garlic, tahini, bell pepper, onion, salt, pepper, and ¼ to ½ cup of water (depending on how thin you want it) and blend on high for about 2 minutes, or until smooth. If the mixture is too thick, add more water, 1 tablespoon at a time, until you reach your desired consistency.

 Cooking tip: This dressing is delicious on just about everything, but especially roasted veggies, salads, and stir-fry dishes.

Per serving (2 tablespoons): Calories: 31; Fat: 3g; Protein: 1g; Carbohydrates: 1g; Fiber: <1g; Sugar: <1g

SOY-FREE

QUICK

ONE POT

NUT-FREE

NO COOK

GLUTEN-FREE

Green Goddess Dressing

Prep time: 10 minutes / Makes ½ cup

SOY-FREE

QUICK

ONE POT

NO COOK

GLUTEN-FREE

2 tablespoons chopped fresh parsley

2 tablespoons chopped fresh basil

1 scallion, green parts only, chopped

1 garlic clove

½ teaspoon salt

½ teaspoon freshly ground black pepper

½ cup tahini

2 tablespoons avocado oil

Juice of 1 lemon

1. In a food processor or high-powered blender, combine the parsley, basil, scallions, garlic, salt, pepper, and ½ cup of water and pulse until pureed.

2. Add the tahini and pulse until combined.

3. Add the avocado oil and lemon juice and pulse again until combined and smooth.

Per serving (2 tablespoons): Calories: 245; Fat: 23g; Protein: 5g; Carbohydrates: 8g; Fiber: 3g; Sugar: 1g

Cilantro Peanut Sauce

Prep time: 5 minutes / Makes 1 cup

QUICK

NO COOK

6 tablespoons peanut butter powder

6 tablespoons warm water

4½ tablespoons low-sodium soy sauce

5 to 6 drops liquid stevia

1½ teaspoons minced fresh ginger

3 teaspoons sesame oil

2 tablespoons minced cilantro

2 teaspoons sesame seeds

1. In a small bowl, whisk together the peanut butter powder and warm water. The peanut butter powder will dissolve as you stir.

2. Add the soy sauce, stevia, ginger, and sesame oil and stir well.

3. Add the cilantro and sesame seeds and stir to combine.

 Love your leftovers: This sauce is extremely versatile and can be used with my Spring Vegetable Rolls with Peanut Sauce (page 76), Loaded Bell Pepper Sandwich (page 69), Cashew and Tofu Stir-Fry (page 88), Green Goddess Buddha Bowl (page 90), and Pad Thai (page 83). Store it in an airtight container in the refrigerator for up to seven days. Shake well before serving.

 Smart shopping: For peanut butter powder, I recommend Better Body Foods brand. You can find powdered peanut butter in the baking aisle.

Per serving (2 tablespoons): Calories: 45; Fat: 3g; Protein: 3g; Carbohydrates: 2g; Fiber: 1g; Sugar: 1g

Not-So-Spicy Jalapeño Hummus

Prep time: 20 minutes, plus 30 minutes to chill / Serves 6

½ cup chopped cilantro

2 jalapeño peppers, seeded and diced

1 garlic clove

3 tablespoons lemon juice

1 (16-ounce) can chickpeas, rinsed, liquid reserved

6 tablespoons tahini

2 tablespoons olive oil

½ teaspoon salt

¼ teaspoon ground cumin

Dash cayenne pepper

1. In a food processor, combine the cilantro, jalapeños, and garlic and pulse until finely chopped.

2. In a medium bowl, mix together the lemon juice and ¼ cup of reserved chickpea water. In another small bowl, mix together the tahini and olive oil and blend well. Set both bowls aside.

3. Add the chickpeas and lemon water to the food processor and puree, scraping down the sides as needed.

4. Add the salt, cumin, cayenne pepper, and tahini mixture and puree until smooth.

5. Transfer the hummus to a bowl, cover it with plastic wrap, and refrigerate it for at least 30 minutes before serving.

 Love your leftovers: The hummus can be easily doubled for a bigger batch and goes with just about any meal in this book. Store it in an airtight container in the refrigerator for up to five days.

Per serving (⅙ cup): Calories: 194; Fat: 14g; Protein: 6g; Carbohydrates: 14g; Fiber: 5g; Sugar: 2g

Homemade Almond Milk

Prep time: 15 minutes / Makes 3 cups

1 or 2 dates, pitted

½ cup raw almonds

1 teaspoon melted
coconut oil

1. Soak 1 or 2 dates (depending on how sweet you want the milk) in a bowl of hot water for 10 minutes.

2. In a high-powered blender, combine the almonds and coconut oil and blend on high for 2 minutes, or until the mixture reaches a nut butter consistency.

3. Add 3 cups of water and the soaked dates and pulse for 1 minute.

4. Store the almond milk in an airtight jar in the refrigerator for up to 7 days. Before serving, give the milk a good stir as separation will occur.

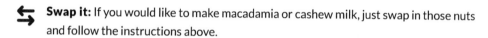 **Swap it:** If you would like to make macadamia or cashew milk, just swap in those nuts and follow the instructions above.

Variation tip: To make chocolate almond milk, add 1 tablespoon of unsweetened cocoa powder and another pitted date to sweeten it up a bit.

Per serving (½ cup): Calories: 73; Fat: 6g; Protein: 2g; Carbohydrates: 3g; Fiber: 1g; Sugar: 1g

SOY-FREE

QUICK

ONE POT

NO COOK

GLUTEN-FREE

5-INGREDIENT

Coconut Yogurt

Prep time: 24 to 32 hours / Cook time: 10 minutes / Makes 2 cups

SOY-FREE

ONE POT

GLUTEN-FREE

5-INGREDIENT

2 (13.5-ounce) cans
full-fat coconut milk

2 tablespoons
tapioca starch

4 probiotic capsules

2 tablespoons maple
syrup (optional)

1. In a medium saucepan over low heat, warm the coconut milk until smooth.

2. Remove ⅓ cup of the warmed coconut milk and place it in a small jar with a lid. Add the tapioca starch and shake well for about 1 minute.

3. Pour the tapioca mixture back into the saucepan, and raise the heat to medium. Bring the coconut milk to a slight simmer and cook, stirring constantly, for about 5 minutes.

4. Remove the coconut milk from the heat and let it cool to 100°F. Add the contents of the probiotic capsules and maple syrup (if using) and stir to combine.

5. Pour the yogurt into sterile glass jars (any size) and cover them with airtight lids. Let the jars sit at room temperature or in a cold oven for 12 to 20 hours. Check on the yogurt occasionally; when it's as thick as you prefer, it is ready.

6. Refrigerate the yogurt for 8 hours before serving. If separation has occurred, just give the yogurt a stir to reconstitute.

7. Serve the yogurt alongside a simple fruit compote or in the Triple Berry Coconut Parfait (page 51).

Cooking tip: If you don't have tapioca starch on hand, other thickeners that can be substituted are chia seeds or agar agar flakes.

 Smart shopping: The probiotic capsules used in this recipe mimic the probiotics in conventional yogurt. It doesn't change the flavor of the yogurt, but it does add some important good bacteria that are especially helpful for your gut. My favorite brand is Culturelle, which can be found at most large retail grocery stores.

Per serving (½ cup): Calories: 320; Fat: 28g; Protein: 3g; Carbohydrates: 8g; Fiber: 0g; Sugar: 5g

White Chocolate Almond Butter

Prep time: 10 minutes / Makes 2 cups

QUICK

ONE POT

NO COOK

GLUTEN-FREE

5-INGREDIENT

2 cups raw almonds

½ cup dairy-free white chocolate chips

½ teaspoon salt

1. In a high-powered blender or food processor, pulse the almonds for 2 to 3 minutes, until they form a paste.

2. Add the white chocolate chips and salt and blend on high for 2 to 3 more minutes, until smooth. If the mixture is too thick, add 1 to 2 tablespoons of water and blend until smooth.

 Love your leftovers: Store the butter in an airtight container in the refrigerator for up to four weeks. This delicious and decadent spread can be used with my Aloha Banana Toast (page 44) and in place of any nut butter; just make sure to keep the amounts the same. Try it out with the sweet version of my French Toast (page 50) in place of cashew butter.

 Smart shopping: For the dairy-free white chocolate chips, I recommend Vegan Sweets or Nestle Toll House.

Variation tip: To change up the flavor of your nut butter, feel free to replace the almonds and white chocolate chips with 2 cups of cashews and ½ cup of vegan dark chocolate chips, and then follow the recipe as instructed.

Per serving (2 tablespoons): Calories: 109; Fat: 9g; Protein: 4g; Carbohydrates: 6g; Fiber: 3g; Sugar: 1g

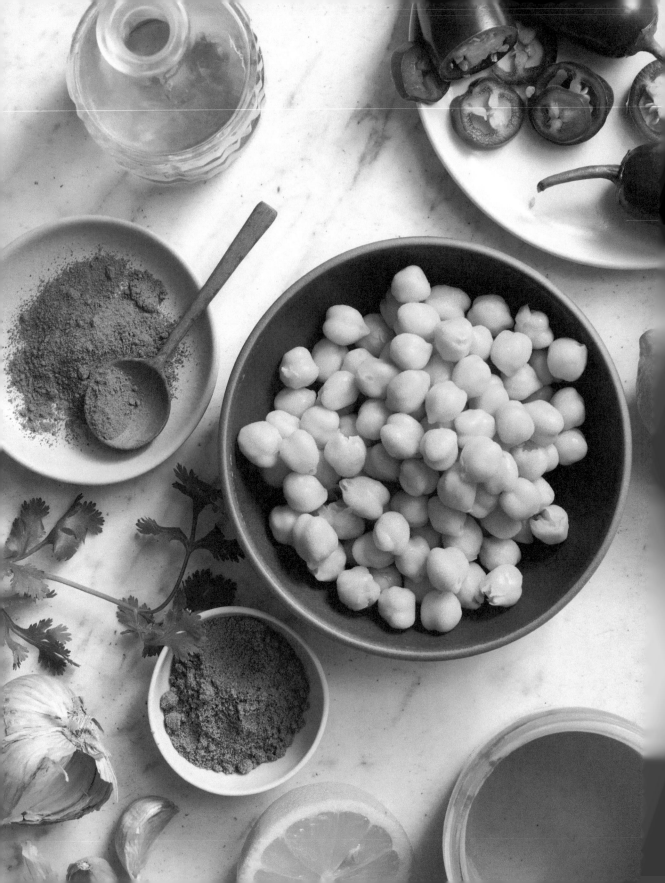

Measurement Conversions

	US STANDARD	US STANDARD (OUNCES)	METRIC (APPROXIMATE)
VOLUME EQUIVALENTS (LIQUID)	2 tablespoons	1 fl. oz.	30 mL
	¼ cup	2 fl. oz.	60 mL
	½ cup	4 fl. oz.	120 mL
	1 cup	8 fl. oz.	240 mL
	1½ cups	12 fl. oz.	355 mL
	2 cups or 1 pint	16 fl. oz.	475 mL
	4 cups or 1 quart	32 fl. oz.	1 L
	1 gallon	128 fl. oz.	4 L
VOLUME EQUIVALENTS (DRY)	⅛ teaspoon		0.5 mL
	¼ teaspoon		1 mL
	½ teaspoon		2 mL
	¾ teaspoon		4 mL
	1 teaspoon		5 mL
	1 tablespoon		15 mL
	¼ cup		59 mL
	⅓ cup		79 mL
	½ cup		118 mL
	⅔ cup		156 mL
	¾ cup		177 mL
	1 cup		235 mL
	2 cups or 1 pint		475 mL
	3 cups		700 mL
	4 cups or 1 quart		1 L
	½ gallon		2 L
	1 gallon		4 L
WEIGHT EQUIVALENTS	½ ounce		15 g
	1 ounce		30 g
	2 ounces		60 g
	4 ounces		115 g
	8 ounces		225 g
	12 ounces		340 g
	16 ounces or 1 pound		455 g
	FAHRENHEIT (F)	**CELSIUS (C) (APPROXIMATE)**	
OVEN TEMPERATURES	250°F	120°C	
	300°F	150°C	
	325°F	180°C	
	375°F	190°C	
	400°F	200°C	
	425°F	220°C	
	450°F	230°C	

References

Centers for Disease Control and Prevention. "Only 1 in 10 Adults Get Enough Fruits or Vegetables." November 16, 2017. CDC.gov/media/releases/2017 /p1116-fruit-vegetable-consumption.html.

Food and Agriculture Organization of the United Nations. *Livestock's Long Shadows: Environmental Issues and Options.* Rome: FAO, 2006. fao.org/3/a0701e /a0701e00.htm.

Forks Over Knives. "The Standard American Diet Is Even Sadder Than We Thought." May 23, 2016. forksoverknives.com/standard-american-diet -sadder-than-we-thought/#gs.vbqjkm.

Home Base (blog). "Reasons Why Eating Breakfast Is Important." August 16, 2017. home-base.co.za/reasons-why-eating-breakfast-is-important.

Petre, Alina. "6 Science-Based Health Benefits of Eating Vegan." *Healthline.* September 23, 2016. healthline.com/nutrition/vegan-diet-benefits#section3.

Petre, Alina. "What Is Veganism, and What Do Vegans Eat?" *Healthline.* August 26, 2019. healthline.com/nutrition/what-is-a-vegan#what-it-is.

Richards, Sarah Elizabeth. "'I Tried Going Vegan for a Week—Here's What Happened." *Women's Health.* December 18, 2017. womenshealthmag.com /food/a19975377/vegan-diet-weight-loss.

Index

G

O

W

Y

Z

Acknowledgments

First and foremost, I would like to thank my editor, Rachel Feldman, for her patience and willingness to work with me. I would also like to give a giant "Thank You" to my husband, Ryan, who has not only encouraged me to live my dream but also made it a reality. Thanks to my children, who have allowed me to sneak away here and there to write, speak, and teach those around me. I hope that one day, you are able to find your passion—and aren't afraid to live it! A big, giant hug to this tribe of believers!

About the Author

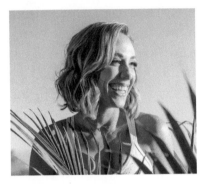

LISA DANIELSON, a.k.a. Veggie Lisa, is a wife of 18 years and a mother of four children ranging in ages from 6 to 15. After tweaking her diet to include more plant-based protein sources, she lost 60 pounds. As a lifelong plant-based eater, she has a passion for vegetables and loves teaching others how delicious vegetables can be! She is an ISSA fitness nutrition specialist, a certified personal trainer, and a corrective exercise specialist. She is the head nutritionist for a major protein supplement company and also helps personal clients reach their weight loss goals. This is her third cookbook. Her motto is: Eat good, feel good, look good!